"MUST BE READ BY ALL PARENTS WHO LOVE THEIR CHILDREN."
—Vincent J. Fontana, M.D., author of *Somewhere a Child Is Crying*

"A valuable guide for health-conscious parents."
—*Booklist*

"Dr. Eden has taken over a very difficult job and his efforts have been successful."
—William H. Weidman, M.D., Mayo Clinic

ALVIN N. EDEN, M.D., is currently Chairman and Director of the Department of Pediatrics at Wyckoff Heights Hospital in Brooklyn and Clinical Associate Professor of Pediatrics, Cornell University Medical College, New York. He is the author of *Positive Parenting* and *Pampers Parents' Handbook*, both available in Signet editions.

ANDREA BOYAR, Ph.D., R.D., is an assistant professor in Dietetics, Food, and Nutrition at Lehman College of the City University of New York and a clinical nutritionist at the American Health Foundation in New York City.

⊘ SIGNET (0451)

PARENTING WISDOM

- ☐ **CHILDRENS MEDICINE: A PARENT'S GUIDE TO PRESCRIPTION AND OVER-THE-COUNTER DRUGS by Ann and James Kepler with Ira Salafsky, M.D.** A clear, concise guide for today's parents faced with a confusing array of prescriptions and over-the-counter drugs for children. With drug profiles, a listing of side effects, cautions and restrictions, and interactions with other drugs, this guide will help you make an informed decision about any trade or generic drug you give your child.
(146549—$3.95)

- ☐ **COPING WITH TEENAGE DEPRESSION, A Parents' Guide by Kathleen McCoy.** Shows parents how to prevent the depression that commonly underlies so-called normal teenage rebellion. There is practical advice on communicating and listening carefully, and on sending out messages of respect and support to troubled young adults. (136632—$4.50)*

- ☐ **DR. EDEN'S HEALTHY KIDS: The Essential Diet, Exercise, and Nutrition Program by Alvin N. Eden, M.D. with Andrea P. Boyar, Ph.D.** Help kids grow up stronger and less vulnerable to such childhood and adulthood health problems as obesity, heart disease, high blood pressure, and diabetes. Solid, accessible information about the kind of diet and exercise that is both healthy and fun. "A valuable guide!"—*Booklist* (160657—$4.95)

- ☐ **SOLO PARENTING: YOUR ESSENTIAL GUIDE *How to Find the Balance Between Parenthood & Personhood* by Kathleen McCoy.** In this comprehensive sourcebook, the author talks with over one hundred solo parents, as well as dozens of professionals, and offers ideas for coping with the tough issues facing single parents. Listings of counseling services, hotline and support organizations. (136632—$4.50)

*Prices slightly higher in Canada

Buy them at your local bookstore or use this convenient coupon for ordering.

NEW AMERICAN LIBRARY
P.O. Box 999, Bergenfield, New Jersey 07621

Please send me the books I have checked above. I am enclosing $_____
(please add $1.00 to this order to cover postage and handling). Send check or money order—no cash or C.O.D.'s. Prices and numbers are subject to change without notice.

Name_____

Address_____

City _____ State _____ Zip Code _____

Allow 4-6 weeks for delivery.
This offer is subject to withdrawal without notice.

DR. EDEN'S HEALTHY KIDS

The Essential Diet, Exercise, and Nutrition Program

by Alvin N. Eden, M.D.,
with Andrea P. Boyar, Ph.D., R.D.

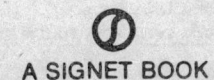

A SIGNET BOOK

NEW AMERICAN LIBRARY

A DIVISION OF PENGUIN BOOKS USA INC.

PUBLISHER'S NOTE

The ideas, procedures, and suggestions contained in this book are not intended as a substitute for consulting with your physician. All matters regarding your child's health require medical supervision.

NAL BOOKS ARE AVAILABLE AT QUANTITY DISCOUNTS WHEN USED TO PROMOTE PRODUCTS OR SERVICES. FOR INFORMATION PLEASE WRITE TO PREMIUM MARKETING DIVISION, NEW AMERICAN LIBRARY, 1633 BROADWAY, NEW YORK, NEW YORK 10019.

Copyright © 1987 by Dr. Alvin N. Eden

Gymboree® Exercises and Games: Copyright © 1987
Gymboree Corporation, Burlingame, California.

All rights reserved

SIGNET TRADEMARK REG. U.S. PAT. OFF. AND FOREIGN COUNTRIES
REGISTERED TRADEMARK—MARCA REGISTRADA
HECHO EN DRESDEN, TN

Dr. Eden's Healthy Kids appeared previously in a Plume edition published by New American Library.

SIGNET, SIGNET CLASSIC, MENTOR, ONYX, PLUME, MERIDIAN and NAL BOOKS are published by New American Library, a division of Penguin Books USA Inc., 1633 Broadway, New York, New York 10019

First Signet Printing, July, 1989

1 2 3 4 5 6 7 8 9

PRINTED IN THE UNITED STATES OF AMERICA

**To Elaine
and to our children, Robert and Elizabeth,
with much love**

Special thanks are due to my secretary, Catherine Hayes. Without her untiring efforts and dedication, it is unlikely that this project could have been completed.

AUTHOR'S NOTE

The English language does not provide any graceful substitute for "he," "she," "his," or "her," so I have again chosen to alternate the pronouns used to describe gender. Please understand that these pronouns refer to your child, even if of the opposite sex, except where I make remarks that apply specifically to girls or boys. I start off Chapter 1 with "she," a decision made not by a flip of a coin but rather because I wanted the chapter on cholesterol and fat to be a "he" chapter, since atherosclerosis is more of a problem for the male.

Contents

FOREWORD   xiii

I. ESSENTIAL FACTS FOR CARING PARENTS
1. It's Up to You   3
2. Emphasize Low-Fat, Low-Cholesterol Foods   10
3. Cut Down on Salt   18
4. Hold the Line on Sugar   23
5. Include Enough Iron   30
6. Add More Fiber   39
7. Fight the S.O.B. Syndrome   43

II. DIET-PLAN MENUS FOR HEALTHIER EATING
8. General Guidelines and Cooking Tips   51
9. Feeding Your Infant   60
10. Feeding Your High-Energy Toddler   70
11. Feeding Your Preschooler   87
12. Feeding Your Active School-ager   103
13. How to Get Your Adolescent to Eat Right   124

III. EXERCISE THAT'S FUN AND EASY
14. Infant Games   165
15. Toddler Activities   177
16. Exercise for Your Preschooler   184
17. Exercise and Sports for Your School-ager   189
18. Exercise and Sports for Your Adolescent   196

IV. NUTRITION FOR THE OVERWEIGHT CHILD

19. Why It's Important to Be Slim — 205
20. Meals for Slimmer Toddlers — 214
21. Feeding the Overweight Preschooler: Just a Stage—or a Problem? — 221
22. Meals for Overweight School-agers — 230
23. Adolescent Obesity: What You Can Do About It — 241

APPENDIX   NUTRITION: THE BASICS   272

Index — 275

Foreword

The task of supervising a child's healthy growth from infancy to young adulthood is a daunting one. Parents must be on constant guard if they are to avoid the pitfalls that await them in guiding their child's nutrition, exercise, and overall physical and emotional well-being.

Am I feeding her the right foods? How can I encourage him to be more active? What about vitamins and supplements? Dr. Alvin Eden knows the answers to the questions parents have about their children's health. Not only that, but he has an excellent track record for making his considerable medical wisdom understandable to parents and their children. In *Dr. Eden's Healthy Kids*, he provides parents with a much-needed guide not only to nutrition and exercise for children, but to building strong health habits now to safeguard them later on in life. *It is the first book devoted to exposing the current epidemic of the unfit child, and the first fitness book for children offering complete low-fat diet plans, nutritional guidelines, and exercise tips.*

I can't disguise the fact that I am a devoted admirer of Dr.

Eden's work, for I am truly aware of the great inroads he has made in teaching fitness and good nutrition to those involved in the health care of infants, children, adolescents, and young adults. Along with his professional expertise, he brings to his work caring concern. Warmth and understanding are the basic ingredients in his gentle attitude toward his patients, and this comes through loud and clear in his writing.

Today, parents are bombarded with all kinds of conflicting information on health and fitness. You need strong guidance and assurance that you are raising your children to be fit and strong. In this wonderful volume, Dr. Eden has attempted to replace the anxiety parents often feel with the knowledge and confidence they need to do the job right. Loving care, patience, and sensitivity are part of the approach. You love your kids, and want them to grow up healthy. Now, in the form of DR. EDEN'S HEALTHY KIDS, you have the power to make it happen.

Lester L. Coleman, M.D.
Medical Columnist, King Features Syndicate

PART I
ESSENTIAL
FACTS FOR
CARING PARENTS

CHAPTER 1

It's Up to You

Is your child really healthy today?
Is she also physically fit and agile?
Does she have strength and stamina?
Does she have a normal blood pressure and a normal or low blood cholesterol level?
Is her weight normal for her age and height?
Does she get sufficient iron?
When you put your child on the Eden Fitness program, your answer to each of these questions will become a confident, resounding "yes"!
Eden is an acronym for:

*E*ssential
*D*iet
*E*xercise
*N*utrition

The fact that my name also happens to be Eden is just a happy coincidence!

AN IMPORTANT ADVANTAGE

The program you are going to discover in this book will give your child an important advantage. It is all about the kind of *diet, exercise,* and *nutrition* that is essential to achieving maximum *fitness* throughout life.

During the thirty years I have been practicing pediatrics, enormous progress has been made in lowering the incidence and even eradicating many serious diseases of childhood. Yet too many of our children remain vulnerable to modern life.

Most kids are just not into fitness. They eat too much of the wrong foods. They rarely get vigorous exercise. Over 30 percent of our kids exhibit at least one of the risk factors associated with heart disease, stroke, or cancer. By age ten, one out of every three children already has an elevated blood cholesterol level, high blood pressure, smokes cigarettes, doesn't exercise sufficiently, or is obese. A high percentage already have heart vessels lined with fatty streaks and plaque—the beginning stages of atherosclerosis or hardening of the arteries. One study has found a 20 percent incidence of significant fatty deposits in the coronary arteries of 15 to 20 year olds! By the end of adolescence many teen-agers already have significant enough degrees of atherosclerosis to put them at extremely high risk of suffering a heart attack or stroke as relatively young adults.

This does not have to happen to your child. I am going to show you how simple changes in childhood diet and exercise can make a big difference later on in life.

Why should we be concerned with children's fitness when heart disease, stroke, obesity, and cancer are adult problems? Why "deprive" our children of the foods all of America is eating with such pleasure when the health problems are decades away? I hope the answers to these two crucial questions will become obvious to you as you read the next few chapters of this book. The two components of the Eden Fitness Program are: 1. the Eden diet plan; 2. the Eden exercise plan.

THE EDEN DIET PLAN: TRY IT FOR SEVEN DAYS

Integral to the Eden Fitness Program is the seven-day diet we've devised for each age group. In just seven days you can put your child on the healthful eating track. The tempting meals and satisfying snacks will help you prove to your child that good food can taste good, too! I'm sure you'll agree that it's worth a week's experiment—and you'll want to continue with variations of your own so that the Eden diet becomes a natural part of your child's life.

Diet patterns start in infancy, continue developing through childhood and adolescence, and solidify in adulthood. The foods we learn to enjoy as children give us psychic pleasure throughout life, whether they are health-promoting or health robbing.

If you had to list the foods that children love most, would you include hamburgers, hot dogs, ice cream, eggs, cheese, fried chicken, pizza, peanut butter, French fries, and chocolate milk shakes? Most parents would. These foods represent the nutritional legacy that is often handed down to our children. But along with this nutritional legacy, we also bequeath something else. We hand down a legacy of serious health problems—obesity, high blood pressure, heart disease, stroke, and cancer.

It seems almost unpatriotic to associate our much-loved national diet with these chronic killer diseases. However, recent scientific evidence points to a definite connection between what we eat, both as children and adults, and what diseases we develop as we age.

The Eden diet plan will help you raise your child in a way that builds good eating habits, not dangerous ones, and leave a legacy for which your children will thank you.

Whether your child is fat or thin or average, one-year old or a fully grown adolescent, it is time to start her on the Eden diet plan. Every child can benefit.

THE EDEN EXERCISE PLAN

The exercise plan of the Eden Fitness Program is easy to follow and fun for everybody. Children do enjoy physical activity and if given half a chance, they will participate with enthusiasm and with increasing skill and endurance. The program does not require Nautilus machines or all sorts of elaborate equipment. The Eden exercise plan encourages increased physical activity of every kind, starting with the infant. It emphasizes and concentrates on developing skills in "carry-over" sports and in aerobic exercises, with specific recommendations and activities appropriate for the age of the child.

This carefully developed, structured, step-by-step program is tailored to the specific activity needs and physical skills of the child, depending on her age and whether or not she is overweight.

Many parents do not realize how important it is to help instill the correct exercise habits in their children. Just as with eating habits, the earlier these patterns are developed the more likely they will continue throughout childhood and, more important, throughout life. There seems to be a general assumption that because kids are basically active they need little or no guidance in developing their physical skills to the fullest or getting enough exercise to stay slim. This simply is not true. Youngsters need direction and encouragement to achieve their maximum fitness potential. Without regular physical activity and the proper exercise no child will develop to the highest level of physical fitness. I do not consider a child really healthy if she is poorly coordinated, flabby, overweight, or if her heart and lungs do not function at peak efficiency. Sad to relate, many studies point to the fact that a high percentage of our preschool, school-age, and adolescent children are indeed physically unfit.

Besides being free of disease, a truly healthy child must be competent to meet her daily tasks, recreational activities and, when a sudden emergency arises, must meet it with maximum vigor and strength. The Eden exercise plan will help make your child healthy in this true sense of the word. She will develop strength, stamina, and endurance and will no longer tire so easily and became exhausted after only a modest amount of physical exertion.

According to the President's Council on Physical Fitness, a 1985 survey of 18,000 grade-school and high-school students showed that:

- 50 percent of girls and 30 percent of boys ages 6 to 12 can't run a mile in less than 10 minutes
- 55 percent of girls ages 6 to 12 can't do one pull-up; 40 percent of boys the same age can do just one
- 40 percent of boys ages 6 to 15 can't reach beyond their toes

BODY IMAGE

Many youngsters grow up with negative feelings about their own bodies, which results in a disturbed and sometimes distorted image of themselves. This inevitably leads to a lowering of self-esteem, self-worth, and self-confidence.

How a person feels about his or her body is very important in terms of emotional stability. The child who is under-exercised becomes flabby, clumsy, and overweight. Such a child does not have enough energy to keep up with his peers. How can you expect such a child to feel good about his body? How can you expect that child to develop a positive body image knowing that he will always be chosen last on the team during gym class?

Sad to relate, many children raised in a sedentary lifestyle look at themselves in the mirror and are very unhappy with what they see. Thus, they start the vicious cycle of depression, binge eating, obesity, and a more and more sedentary lifestyle.

GROWING UP FIT

You are about to increase your child's chances of living a longer, happier life. The program you are going to discover in this book will give your child an important advantage in achieving maximum fitness throughout life.

The EDEN Program will give you the means to direct your child's eating and exercise habits so that he or she grows up fit today and less vulnerable to serious illness in the future. I can't promise any child the Garden of Eden. But I can promise that she has a far better chance of becoming a healthier and stronger adult if you take charge of her health right now.

Any parent who cares enough about a child's health, however, can break that vicious cycle—or keep it from starting in the first place.

YOUR ESSENTIAL GUIDELINES

The best way to put your child on the road to lifetime fitness can be summed up with six simple guidelines:

1. *Emphasize Low-Fat, Low-Cholesterol Foods.* Getting into the low-fat, low-cholesterol habit will give your child a head start on fighting hardening of the arteries and heart disease later on in life.
2. *Cut Down on Salt.* If your child learns to enjoy less salty foods now, chances are he'll continue with a low-salt diet later on, when high-salt intake and high blood pressure are linked.
3. *Hold the Line on Sugar.* Curb a sweet tooth to make sure your child is getting enough of the basic nutrients found in nonsugary foods—and fighting obesity.
4. *Include Enough Iron.* An iron-rich diet can prevent fatigue, misbehavior, and anemia.
5. *Add More Fiber.* Not only will fiber aid digestion, but there's evidence that it will help protect your child against a number of gastrointestinal diseases including appendicitis, diverticulitis, and cancer of the colon and rectum in adulthood.
6. *Fight the S.O.B. Syndrome.* If you encourage your child to exercise instead of watching T.V. (the "sitting-on-behind" syndrome), he'll carry good exercise habits with him through life, and protect himself from

ailments such as heart disease, high blood pressure, and obesity.

The next few chapters will explain the research and experience behind these guidelines. Once you see how important they are, I'm sure you will be as confident as I am that the Eden Fitness Program is well worth trying.

CHAPTER 2
Emphasize Low-Fat, Low-Cholesterol Foods

Most children eat lots of fatty red meats, too many eggs, and loads of fried foods. They also drink large quantities of whole milk. The common denominator of this typical diet is its high animal fat content, which leads to high levels of cholesterol in the blood. Elevated blood cholesterol levels are associated with the formation of plaque (which has cholesterol as its major ingredient) in the arteries. When arterial plaque, the plaque on the inner walls of the arteries leading to the heart, becomes thick enough, it can obstruct the blood flow to the heart, and the result is a heart attack or myocardial infarction.

"But toddlers don't have heart attacks," many parents counter when I discuss the reasons for my concern about their children's high-fat/high cholesterol diets. They're right of course. Toddlers don't develop enough hardening of the arteries to cause a heart attack. However, tracking studies, in which children are tested at intervals over a number of years, indicate that blood cholesterol levels increase with advancing age. The toddler who tests high in blood cholesterol at age three has been found to have an even higher blood cholesterol level when rechecked at age ten.

"I have rarely started to think about heart disease myself because I am still under thirty," a young father recently said to me. "And now, Dr. Eden, you're telling me that I should already be concerned about my two year old." Let me assure you that now is the best time to be concerned.

Like many other young parents this father believed that his relative "youth" protected him from heart disease. He thought he had at least a good ten years or so to go before there was any need for him to think seriously about his own risk of developing atherosclerosis—the medical term for hardening of the arteries. The idea that he could and *should* act now not only to protect himself but to protect his child came as a complete shock. Perhaps you're surprised, too. This chapter should make it clear, however, that you'll be giving your child tremendous health advantages with the Eden Fitness Program.

Clearly, preventing blood cholesterol levels from rising is one of the most important things a parent can do to protect a child from suffering from coronary heart disease later on in life. The best way to keep your child's cholesterol level at a safe level is to offer him a low-fat, low-cholesterol diet starting now.

CRUCIAL AMERICAN HEART ASSOCIATION RECOMMENDATIONS

Dr. Ronald Lauer, the Director of the Division of Pediatric Cardiology at the University of Iowa School of Medicine, said in 1980, "Although we do not have proof that a prudent diet for all children will slow down atherosclerosis, it makes intuitive sense for this to be done now." At that time I wrote: "I agree completely with Dr. Lauer and hope that the American Heart Association will officially come out with this recommendation shortly."

In June 1983 the American Heart Association officially published their recommendation stating that all healthy children over the age of two years should be fed a diet in which: (1) total fat should be about 30 percent of the calories, 10 percent or less from saturated fat; (2) total daily cholesterol intake should not exceed 300 milligrams.

Quoting from the summary of this American Heart Association recommendation: "Physicians who care for the young have a unique and important role in reducing the incidence of the complications of atherosclerosis in adults through the installation of preventive measures in childhood. The use of a prudent diet, reduced in fat content in healthy children is a safe and most likely effective way to achieve an important element of these preventive measures."

I believe that the year between a toddler's first and second birthday is also crucial. Instead of waiting this whole year during which the toddler will eat all the high-fat, high-cholesterol foods that are typical in the American diet, why not start immediately after the child is switched to table food? Why allow bad habits to take hold at all? Why take the chance that undesirable food preferences will develop? Why not take advantage of the fact that during this year your control over what your child eats is greater than it ever will be again?

As Dr. Robert Levy, the former Director to the Heart, Lung and Blood Institute has stated: "There is every reason to believe that prevention should begin early when the child begins to eat regular foods."

THE CHOLESTEROL FACTOR

Many studies of school-aged children have proven that diet modification can lower blood cholesterol levels. In one boarding school study the children were put on a low cholesterol, low fat diet for just six weeks and their average blood cholesterol levels were lowered by 10%. A modest change in diet over a number of months can lower cholesterol levels by as much as 25%.

In 1984, the American Health Foundation sponsored a symposium that brought together 37 heart specialists to discuss the problem of cholesterol and diet in children. Their concluding statement included the following points:

1. The average blood cholesterol level of children in the United States is too high (average of 160 milligrams percent).
2. Children's blood cholesterol levels should be lowered in order to reduce the risk of heart attacks later on in life.

3. A healthy diet for children should be low in cholesterol and in saturated fat.
4. The two main problems in current children's diets are excessive consumption of red meats and whole milk products.
5. Elevated blood cholesterol levels in children lead to elevated blood cholesterol levels in adults.

AMERICAN CANCER SOCIETY AGREES

There is another important reason to reduce the amount of fat in your child's diet and that is its relationship to cancer. The American Cancer Society recommends that high fiber, fruits, vegetables and whole grain cereals be substituted for many fatty foods. There appears to be an increased incidence of cancer of the breast, colon and prostate in people who eat high fat diets. For example, in Japan where the diet is low in fat, the incidence of breast cancer is low. While it is true that these cancers are not seen in children, the point to remember is that children who become accustomed to high fat diets are much more likely to continue eating the same way as adults and then their chances of developing one of these cancers will increase.

THE LIPOPROTEIN FACTOR

In recent years we have learned a great deal about the importance of cholesterol-lipoproteins as they relate to the development of atherosclerosis. There are two main types of lipoprotein, low-density lipoprotein (LDL) and high-density lipoprotein (HDL). About 75 percent of the total cholesterol is contained within LDL and about 25 percent is in HDL. The LDL have been found to carry cholesterol from the blood to the tissues to be deposited on the arterial walls. This can lead to the development of cholesterol plaque and atherosclerosis. Because of this function LDL has been labeled the "bad" lipoprotein. On the other hand, HDL has been called the "good" lipoprotein because it has been found to clean and vacuum out the blood vessel walls by carrying cholesterol away to the liver, where it is processed and excreted from the body. It is obvious from all this that it would be ideal to reduce the blood level of the "bad" LDL and to raise the level of the "good" HDL in order to protect against developing atherosclerosis. To a large extent this can be accomplished with proper diet and exercise.

"GOOD" FATS AND "BAD" FATS

What is the role of dietary fat in developing atherosclerosis? Here again there are "good" fats and "bad" fats. The "good" fats are the polyunsaturated fats, such as liquid vegetable oils made from corn, safflower, sunflower, and soybeans, which have been shown to lower blood cholesterol levels. There is some evidence that these polyunsaturated fats may also lower the level of the "bad" LDL's. Another group of "good" fats includes certain long-chain fatty acids found in fish, such as tuna, salmon, and sardines. It has been found that these fatty acids also help lower blood cholesterol levels. The "bad" fat in terms of atherosclerosis is saturated fat. A diet high in saturated fat consistently raises blood cholesterol levels. In fact, some investigators believe that saturated fat is a much more important cause of high blood cholesterol levels than a high-cholesterol diet. Saturated fats are those fats that are hard at room temperature, as opposed to the polyunsaturated fats that are liquid at room temperature. Among the foods that are high in saturated fats are beef, pork, whole milk, ice cream, vegetable shortenings, and palm and cocoanut oil, both used in processed foods.

HIGH-FAT, HIGH-CHOLESTEROL FOODS KIDS LIKE

High-Fat Foods	*Portion Size*	*Fat (grams)*
Butter	1 teaspoon	4
Margarine	1 teaspoon	4
Mayonnaise	1 tablespoon	12

HIGH-FAT, HIGH-CHOLESTEROL FOODS KIDS LIKE

High-Fat Foods	Portion Size	Fat (grams)
Salad dressings	2 tablespoons	12
French fries	½ cup	12
Hamburger—medium fat, cooked	3 oz. patty	15
Hot dog	1 (8/lb.)	15
Lamb chop (lean and fat)	3 oz.	17
Cheese, hard	1 ounce	10
Macaroni and cheese	1 cup	22
Peanuts	½ cup	35
Whole milk	1 cup	8
Cream cheese	1 tablespoon	5
Vegetable oil	1 tablespoon	15
Peanut butter	1 tablespoon	10
Ice cream	1 cup	14

High-Cholesterol Foods	Portion Size	Cholesterol (milligrams) (rounded to nearest zero or 5)
Egg—large	1 yolk	275
Hamburger	Quarter pounder	70
Liver	4 ounces	400
Ice cream	1 cup	55–85
Custard—baked	4 ounces	105
Shrimp	1 cup	200
Chicken à la king	1 cup	185
Sponge cake	1 piece	123
Cream puffs with custard	Average	150
Ice cream—French vanilla, soft serve	1 cup	155
Pies: Lemon chiffon	Serving	180
Custard	Serving	160
Lemon meringue	Serving	130
Fried chicken—Kentucky	3½ ounce	115–135
McDonald's scrambled eggs	Serving	300

THE BOTTOM LINE

During the past twenty years the average adult blood cholesterol level in the United States has been lowered. The average American adult has decreased his intake of foods rich in saturated fat and increased his intake of polyunsaturated fats, especially polyunsaturated vegetable oils. These dietary modifications have also been associated with a decrease in the death rate from atherosclerosis. Butter consumption has dropped 30 percent, eggs 14 percent, animal fats 60 percent, and deaths from heart disease dropped about 30 percent.

During this same twenty-year period, however, there has been little, if any, change in the diets of our children. Why?

Dr. Eugene Passani, Associate Director of Cardiology at the National Institute of Health, recently explained: "Most physicians are used to treating acute illnesses. They are less comfortable with preventive medicine for healthy looking patients. Few doctors recommend dietary reform to a patient unless the cholesterol level is elevated or he has suffered a heart attack." This statement helps explain why so many pediatricians do not forcefully advocate significant dietary changes for all healthy children. I cannot accept this "laissez-faire" attitude, however. Pediatricians have always been in the forefront in terms of prevention. Preventing heart attacks and strokes is at least as important as preventing polio and diphtheria.

Another reason some members of the pediatric community do not advocate significant diet modification for all children is that there has not been any *direct* demonstration by controlled studies that dietary changes during childhood will lower the incidence of coronary artery disease later on in life. While this is true, my answer to these skeptics is that it is very unlikely that we will ever have this type of cause-and-effect evidence from controlled studies. This dispute reminds me of the argument about the relationship between cigarette smoking and lung cancer. The tobacco industry continues to insist that there is no direct evidence from properly controlled studies proving that cigarette smoking directly causes lung cancer. They call for more studies. Tobacco industry spokespeople suggest that perhaps the increased incidence of lung cancer in recent years may be related to some factor other than cigarettes. Are they referring to more bathtubs or television sets as causing more lung cancer? Obviously, this is utter and complete nonsense.

THE EDEN LOW-FAT, LOW-CHOLESTEROL ADVANTAGE

The Eden Fitness Program will help your child get into the low-fat habit because it sticks to these cholesterol- and fat-fighting rules:

- It will reduce your child's total fat intake to 30 percent or less of his total daily calories, with 10 percent or less of these calories from saturated fat.
- It will reduce his total cholesterol intake per day to less than 300 milligrams.
- It will get him to exercise—sustained physical activity helps sweep cholesterol away from the artery walls.
- Is he obese? If so, the Eden Fitness Program will help him slim down. If not, it will keep him trim. Remember—obesity and high cholesterol levels often go hand in hand.

I am convinced that the prevention of atherosclerosis rests in large measure with *never* allowing cholesterol levels to rise to dangerous levels. The Eden Fitness Program does the job with no known down-side risk.

CHAPTER 3
Cut Down on Salt

When I told the father of one of my young patients it would be better if his family ate less salt, he protested. "But Doctor," he said, "we hardly ever eat pretzels or potato chips or olives." He knew those three foods have a high salt content, but apparently he was unaware of how much of this potentially dangerous substance is contained in other items as well. "Do you put a lot of catsup on your meat at your house?" I asked him. "Are canned vegetables and soups, bacon, oil-packed tuna, pickles, lunch meats, pizza, frequently served?" His answers were all in the affirmative, and eventually I was able to make my point. Salt is an insidious ingredient in many of the foods we eat. On top of that (literally!) more salt is added at the table.

I am happy to report that most children quickly adjust to the taste of food without added salt. Six-year-old Margaret's mother, for example, told me that when she first began to cut down on salt in cooking, her daughter commented several times that the food "tasted funny." This did not deter her from continuing the low-salt cooking. Six months later, during a visit to an aunt's house, Margaret whispered to her mother that the food tasted funny. "In what way?" asked the mother. "Too salty," was the reply.

The average daily intake of salt in the United States is 10–15 grams or between 2 and 2½ teaspoons, and this is many times what the body requires. The safe and adequate requirements of salt are estimated to be between 1–3 grams per day. About one-third of the daily salt intake comes from the naturally-occurring salt in foods, one-third is added during cooking and with the use of the salt shaker during the meal, and the final one-third comes from the salt that is added during commercial processing.

Does too much salt inevitably lead to high blood pressure? The answer clearly is no. *Everyone* who eats the standard American diet, which is much too high in salt, doesn't become hypertensive. We have not yet discovered all the factors that make one person who eats too much salt hypertensive, whereas another person who eats the same amount isn't.

In the meantime, why take chances? It is relatively easy to cut back on salt simply by avoiding the foods with high salt content and using as little salt as possible during cooking.

"But, Dr. Eden, why should I worry about Peter having a heart attack or stroke or kidney failure from high blood pressure? After all, he's only five." I have to concede the point, but my concern is not that the preschooler will suffer one of these catastrophes or even that he is likely to develop high blood pressure during his preschool years (although it is worth noting that a small percentage of young children already *do* have high blood pressure). Rather, I worry that Peter's diet is much too high in salt and if he continues to eat the same way, he will be at greater risk to develop hypertension later on in life.

HIGH SODIUM FOODS TO CUT DOWN ON

Catsup
Bacon
Canned meats and canned vegetables
Frankfurters
Certain shellfish (crab, lobster, and shrimp)
Soy sauce
Boullion cubes
Pickles and relishes
Salted popcorn, pretzels, and nuts

Ground beef and ham
Luncheon meats
Tomato sauce
Canned tuna in oil
Fast-food hamburgers, chicken, and pizza
Canned vegetable soups

SALT AND HIGH BLOOD PRESSURE

Hypertension is connected with heart attack, stroke, and kidney failure. Although a cause-and-effect relationship between a high-salt intake and hypertension has not been established, studies done in many countries around the world clearly indicate that in populations where salt consumption is high, so is the incidence of hypertension. One out of eight adults in the United States suffers from high blood pressure. Conversely, in populations that have low salt intakes, there is much less hypertension.

You are probably wondering what hypertension and its possible complications have to do with children. For one thing, starting in infancy blood pressure starts to rise and continues to rise with increasing age. For another, some school-age children already have high blood pressure. Additionally, there is evidence that children who eat large quantities of salt have the greatest rise in blood pressure over the years. Because of all this, I and many other pediatricians and public health officials believe that limiting salt during childhood is one way to keep blood pressure from climbing too high later on.

In primitive societies in remote areas of the world, such as the Kallahari Bushmen of South Africa and the Melesian tribes of New Guinea, daily sodium intake is low and high blood pressure is rarely found. Furthermore, their blood pressures do not rise with advancing age as they do in technologically advanced societies such as our own. It is estimated that in Japan about 1 teaspoon of soy sauce—which is high in sodium—is eaten per meal. Not surprisingly, the leading health problem in Japan today is high blood pressure and strokes. Further support for the relationship between sodium intake and high blood pressure comes from various migration studies. When primitive societies move and adopt more modern ways of life, including increased salt intake, their blood pressures promptly and dramatically rise.

There has been some fascinating research related to the blood pressure readings of the Qush'kua mountain nomads of southern Iran. These people, despite lean bodies and hard physical labor, both of which usually keep blood pressures down, have in fact a high incidence of hypertension (about 15 percent of their population). One reasonable explanation is their diet—which turns out to be extremely high in salt.

Can high blood pressure be *prevented* by starting a baby on a controlled salt intake diet and maintaining that diet throughout childhood and into adult life? We don't know for sure, but there is some evidence suggesting that the answer is yes. An interesting study published in the July 1983 issue of the *Journal of the American Medical Association*, supports the case for a low-salt diet preventing the subsequent development of high blood pressure. Doctor Albert Hofman and his colleagues at Erasmus University Medical School, Rotterdam, The Netherlands, performed a double-blind study with 476 newborns. They were divided into two groups—one group was put on a regular normal salt diet and the other group was put on a low-salt diet. Blood pressure was carefully monitored throughout the six months of the study. By six months of age, the average systolic blood pressure of the low-salt group babies was lower than the systolic blood pressures in the group fed a normal salt diet. Quoting from the conclusion of this investigation, "These findings support the view that sodium intake is closely related to the level of blood pressure. Moderation of sodium intake starting from early in life might perhaps contribute to the prevention of high blood pressure and of rise in blood pressure with age."

Doctor Beverly Morgan, Professor and Chairman of the Department of Pediatrics at the University of California, Ervine, College of Medicine, lectured to the Los Angeles Pediatric Society on the subject of childhood hypertension. She believes that the evidence to date is sufficient to justify the recommendation of a modest sodium restriction for all children, whether or not they have high blood pressure. Doctor R. Curtis Allison, the

Director of the Division of Pediatric Cardiology of the Children's Medical Center, Harvard Medical School and an authority on childhood hypertension, writes: "It is certainly reasonable to advise a low sodium diet from birth for a healthy infant. If the sodium intake is maintained at a low level throughout life, hypertension will be prevented." I agree with both these experts. The best way to prevent the onset of hypertension in childhood and later on during adult life is to cut down on salt intake right from the start.

THE EDEN LOW-SODIUM ADVANTAGE

The Eden diet plan is low in salt. Unlike the craving for sugar, which may indeed be genetically determined, the craving and need for extra salt beyond the natural salt content in foods is acquired after birth. Studies have shown that newborn infants are indifferent to salty-tasting solutions. In my experience, babies who are raised on a low sodium diet are happy with the taste of the foods they eat. Many parents make the mistake of tasting their baby's food first and seasoning it to their own taste before offering it to the child. This is a mistake. If you don't add extra salt to the baby food, he will not acquire a taste for salty foods. As early as six months of age a baby who has been fed foods with added salt will refuse to eat nonsalty foods. Other investigations have shown that a preference for salt clearly exists in preschool-age children.

Believe me, when a taste for excessive salt becomes established, it is a hard one to deal with. When I was very young my mother used to bribe me with olives and pickles rather than with high-sugar treats. Don't ask me why—she just did. To this day my taste buds cry out for salty foods, not sugar. Resisting is a terrible struggle.

On the Eden diet plan a low-salt diet is provided. If you begin using the plan early on, an intense craving for salt is less likely to develop as your child grows older.

CHAPTER 4
Hold the Line on Sugar

"I know my Sally should be eating fewer sweets but she's just like me—born with a sweet tooth," exclaimed the mother of an overweight four year old. She was not the first mother I have met who seemed to believe that her child's desire for sweets was congenital. And she certainly won't be the last. Actually, the theory that people are born with a craving for sweet is a plausible one.

We are a nation of sweet-tooths. According to recent figures from the U.S. Department of Agriculture the average consumption of sugar per person is over 120 pounds per year. Almost 20 percent of our total daily calories comes from sweeteners added to foods, such as sugar, honey, and corn syrup. These numbers clearly show that most of us, including our children, eat far much too much sugar.

The craving for sweets has a long history. A painting found in a cave in southern Spain, estimated to be 20,000 years old, showed a Neolithic man stealing honey from a beehive. There is one theory that proposes that sweets were used by early man as an indicator in food selection, because at that time most sweet-tasting foods were safe to eat.

Why do we eat so much sugar? Why do children enjoy sweet-tasting foods? Why is it so difficult to get a child to cut down on his daily intake of sweets? We are not certain, but there is strong evidence that the human desire for sweet-tasting foods is innate. Studies have shown that taste buds are already present and functioning in four-month-old fetuses. At five months of fetal life the swallowing rate increases after a sweet stimulus has been injected into the amniotic sac. A number of investigations have demonstrated that newborns exhibit positive responses to sweet solutions but are indifferent to salty solutions. It is significant that the first food that many newborns consume, namely, breast milk, is relatively sweet to the taste.

Although the taste for sweetness may be genetic, the taste for overly sweetened foods is definitely acquired. A good example of this is the fact that almost all infants will drink water that has not been sweetened. If an infant is offered water with added sugar however, she will then usually refuse to drink unsweetened water after that. The point is that it is very easy for a baby to develop a taste for overly sweetened foods. If you make sure that sugar is not added to your infant's water or to her solid foods, she will be much less likely to grow up craving and devouring excess quantities of sugar.

Another reason that many children eat large amounts of sugar-laden foods is the early association between this kind of food and good behavior. It has been my experience that parents often use food as a reward or as a soother of hurt feelings. Have any of us as children not been offered a cookie or a lollipop to stop crying? Sweet foods are often associated with pleasing a parent. How many toddlers have been told, "If you behave yourself I will give you a piece of chocolate"? Sugar-rich foods often become associated with love. "If you love your mother you'll finish all your vegetables—and then I'll give you some cookies."

Finally, children associate overly sweet foods with happy times, such as parties and outings. The result of all this is that the genetic inborn preference for mildly sweet-tasting foods changes during early childhood into an acquired taste for overly sweetened foods, and this craving for sweets becomes difficult to control.

Sweet substances come in many forms. Sugar is the general term for a carbohydrate that tastes sweet. White table sugar or sucrose is not a natural food but rather a highly refined processed product that is made from sugar beets and sugar cane. Brown sugar is white sugar whose surface has been sprayed with very small amounts of molasses. Lactose is the sugar that is found in milk. Honey is a rich, pleasant-tasting sweetener that consists primarily of fructose, the fruit sugar that is also naturally found in fruit juices. It has a better reputation than white table sugar, but doesn't offer any more nutrition. Honey has 65 calories per tablespoon, whereas sucrose (white table sugar) and lactose have 45 calories per tablespoon. Molasses is a by-product of sucrose production, and has a very strong sweet taste. It is a source of iron and calcium and so has more nutritional value than either table sugar or honey. Molasses can add an interesting flavor to certain foods such as bran muffins, gingersnaps, and Indian pudding. Sugar (except for molasses) contributes nothing but calories to a child's diet and it *replaces* other sources of essential nutrients. Sugar contains *no* nutrients—that is, no vitamins or minerals or fiber, no protein or essential fats. It provides simple, refined processed carbohydrate that is not essential to well-being and is devoid of health-giving properties.

The key to understanding why too much sugar is unhealthy for children (and also for adults) is the concept of nutrient density. Let's consider a child who eats about 2,000 calories per day. Within this caloric allowance, the foods she consumes should contain essential nutrients—vitamins and minerals, essential fatty acids, amino acids, complex carbohydrates, and fiber. The greater the number of calories that are "empty" (i.e., lacking in essential nutrients), the more likely the total diet will not supply all her needed nutrients. Marginal nutritional deficiencies develop in those children who eat too many "empty" sugar calories each day. Candy, for example, is composed almost entirely of refined sugar. Soft drinks are sugar-water mixtures. Even though flour and shortening are used in addition to sugar in cakes and cookies, these ingredients add very little in the way of nutrition. Thus we call the calories supplied by most highly sweetened foods, "empty calories." High sugar intake often means high intake of calories, and a high calorie diet leads to obesity. Because highly sweetened foods taste so good, children have a tendency to eat large amounts and so take in huge numbers of calories. I suppose there is some child somewhere who does not respond positively to the taste of candy, cake, cookies, ice cream, and such, but I haven't found her yet.

There have been a number of well-publicized claims that high sugar diets in children can lead to hyperactivity. The consensus, however, based on carefully controlled studies, is that there is *no* relationship between excessive sugar intake and hyperactivity.

As a seasoning, sugar in small quantities is useful in making some foods more appealing to children. A small amount of sugar added to oatmeal may make an initially unappealing cereal that much more desirable. The end result is that the child now will eat a very nutritious breakfast which she otherwise would have refused. A bit of jam spread on whole-wheat bread or some sugar sprinkled on cut strawberries are other examples of this principle. Fiber, complex carbohydrates, vitamins A, C, folic acid, and potassium are thus supplied to a child who might otherwise refuse the bread or fruit without the sweetener.

In addition to obesity, there are a number of other health problems associated with the excessive consumption of sugar, and these problems can begin early in life. For starters, sugar is not beneficial for your child's teeth. This is not exactly earth-shattering news. In fact, I bet that there isn't one single parent reading this who does not know of the relationship between sugar and tooth decay. Yet I find that there is often remarkably little concern displayed with regard to the toddler's teeth. "They're only her baby teeth, and she won't have them for long," is the usual justification I hear for this lackadaisical attitude. "When she gets her permanent teeth, we will be more careful about limiting sweets."

No one can argue with the fact that baby teeth are not permanent, but they're still important. I have seen two year olds whose front teeth had to be removed because they were so badly decayed from taking a bottle of juice, sweetened water, or milk to bed each night. Without those front teeth, chewing becomes more difficult for the toddler, and biting into anything crispy or crunchy is almost impossible. I have also seen three year olds with ten or more fillings in their teeth. Although it is true that fluoride is very important in preventing teeth decay, and some children are born with teeth that are more vulnerable to decay than others, sugar is the catalyst, and it is highly unlikely that there would have been as *many* cavities had these kids been given fewer high-sugar foods.

"It seems a little late to cut down on sugar. My son already has a mouthful of cavities," the father of a nine year old answered when I urged him to modify Frank's diet. He was right. Something should have been done earlier, but as somebody once said, better late than never. I also pointed out that his son will have a lot more cavities in the future if he continues to eat so much sugar. I concluded my lecture by reminding him that the only one who will benefit by a continuing laissez-faire attitude about the sugar in Frank's diet was his dentist. "If my daughter refuses to quit loading up on candy, at least let her start paying her own dental bills," said the father of a sixteen year old, with a wry grin.

Much of the problem of dental caries can be *prevented* through good dental hygiene (including adequate amounts of fluoride) and a proper diet, one that is limited in foods that contain large amounts of refined sugar. Even if your child already has a mouthful of cavities it's still not too late to try to help her save many good teeth. We tend to think of tooth decay as a disease primarily of childhood but the truth of the matter is that cavities continue to develop throughout life if diet and dental hygiene remain poor. Besides regular visits to the dentist, fluoride and instruction in proper brushing and flossing of teeth, reducing the sugar content of meals and snacks served at home will prevent or slow further deterioration of the teeth.

Another potential danger of excessive sugar intake is the evidence that it may, in some cases, predispose to elevated blood fat levels, a risk factor for heart disease and stroke later on in life. About 10 percent of the population responds to a high sugar intake this way.

Your efforts to limit the sugar in your child's diet should be focused on the foods she eats at home. Obviously that means that high-sugar, high-calorie, low-nutrition desserts must cease to be the "pièce de résistance" at the end of every family dinner. I am not suggesting that cake or pie never should appear on the table, only that cake or pie should be considered special treats to be served on special occasions only. I remember one mother looking grief stricken when I told her how important it was to stop serving fancy desserts. She explained that she and her eight-year-old Kristen spent many pleasant hours together baking and decorating cakes. "I don't want to give up the closeness we share when we bake together." This was a tough one, because I am a firm believer in parent/child happy sharing of activities. As I was trying to think of an appropriate answer, Mrs. S. brightened almost immediately and said, "I know, I will teach Kristen how to knit. It will be a way of still spending time together and it will be healthier for both of us." Hers was a much better solution than I could have thought of.

If you want to give your child all the benefits of good nutrition but unfortunately you are a sugar freak, it is time to get a grip on yourself. It is unrealistic to expect a young child not to want the treats she sees her parents eating. To do right by your little one, you will have to set the right example. Think of it this way: If you don't *buy* high sugar treats, they won't be there in the cupboard to tempt you. You won't be able to eat them and neither will your child. You are all better off. (Nobody ever said being a parent was easy.)

Obviously, if you have been using high-sugar treats as rewards, you must stop. There are lots of better ways to reward your child than with food. Hugs and kisses are much more appropriate to show your love and approval. A temporary withdrawal of a privilege is a more effective means of showing your disapproval than cutting out a sugar-filled treat.

THE EDEN LOW SUGAR ADVANTAGE

You can expect some loud complaints if your child is already a sugar freak, but the Eden diet plan will help you stick to your guns when you offer fruits, raw vegetables, or yogurt instead of cookies or cakes at snack time. You'll start to replace sugar-laden treats with fruit for dessert as often as possible. Whole-grain muffins, cereals, and fruit juices will eventually substitute for sweet bakery products, sugared cereals, and soft drinks. If at first your child refuses to eat the new healthy snacks or looks with disgust at the fruit for dessert, don't worry about it, and above all don't give in. You may not believe it, but in time she will start eating and enjoying these foods.

The occasional sweet on special occasions is fine. It is a mistake to be fanatic about the monitoring of every single food item that your child picks up. Not only that, I think it would be unrealistic and unnecessarily harsh to attempt to impose an absolute no-sugar policy on your child.

CHAPTER 5
Include Enough Iron

At this moment, hundreds of thousands, perhaps millions of American children may be suffering from iron-poor diets. The consequences of a diet too low in iron range from fatigue to misbehavior to intellectual slowness. These children may also have trouble in concentrating and often show little interest in the world around them. These signs and symptoms obviously don't always signal iron deficiency, but rather could be related to any number of other causes. Yet, iron deficiency should always be a prime suspect.

When I asked the father of fourteen-year-old Jordan whether his son ate iron-rich vegetables, liver, iron-fortified cereal, or took an iron supplement, the answer was no. But he assured me his son had recently been tested and was found not to be anemic. This father thought that if Jordan was not anemic, he could not possibly be suffering from iron deficiency.

I had to explain to him that recent research on the subject indicates that iron deficiency can indeed be a problem even when anemia is not present. This is news to many parents and so is the fact that the symptoms of iron deficiency, with or without anemia, can include lethargy, behavior disturbances, and decreased intellectual ability.

During the past few years we have learned that iron deficiency is a much more significant problem than just a common cause of anemia. As a matter of fact, some investigators in this field believe that the anemia of iron deficiency is relatively unimportant unless it is very severe. Doctor Frank Oski, Chairman of the Department of Pediatrics, Johns Hopkins School of Medicine, a well-respected authority on the subject, wrote in a recent article in the *American Journal of Diseases of Children*, "The actual anemia caused by iron deficiency is the least important manifestation of this heavy metal deficiency."

There is now enough evidence to conclude that iron deficiency is a systemic disease that may have harmful effects on many organ systems of the body. Of greatest significance to pediatricians and to parents is the recent data implicating iron deficiency as a cause of *learning problems* in youngsters. Lack of iron can adversely affect both the *behavior* and the *intellectual* development of infants and children. A number of investigations with preschool-aged children have shown that iron deficiency causes shortened attention span, disruptive behavior, lack of cooperation, and poor mental performance. There is little question that iron deficiency, even without the anemia, can result in biochemical alterations in the body, which impair behavior and performance in infants and children.

Iron is a basic essential chemical element that cannot be manufactured by the body. It must be provided either in the foods we eat or as a supplement in concentrated form. In order to maintain optimal good health, both physical and intellectual, a continuous daily supply of iron is needed. Iron is indirectly related to the red blood cells, specifically to the oxygen-carrying pigment of the red blood cell called hemoglobin. Hemoglobin is a complex molecule made up of heme and globin. Each unit of heme requires an atom of iron and so in order for the body to produce adequate amounts of hemoglobin it must be provided with a steady supply of iron. This is essential because of the important role that hemoglobin plays in supplying oxygen to the body and brain. Anemia develops when the hemoglobin level in the blood drops below a certain level (below 12 gm/dl). At any given time, we are either iron sufficient or iron deficient. An iron-deficient state develops when the iron intake is insufficient to meet the body's needs or when excessive bleeding occurs.

The great majority of cases of iron deficiency result from faulty eating habits—when the daily diet does not supply enough iron.

The simplest way to understand iron metabolism is to realize that every one of us falls into one of three different categories:

1. *Iron sufficiency*, meaning that the body has adequate iron stores for all its requirements.
2. *Iron deficiency without anemia*. This is an extremely important and relatively new concept. In this state the person has not yet become anemic because of inadequate iron intake, but is still iron deficient because there is not enough stored iron to satisfy all the body's needs. Besides its role as a component of hemoglobin, iron is also a structural part of enzymes that are critical in metabolism, DNA synthesis, and neurotransmitter synthesis. Because of this vital role in brain function, iron deficiency, even without the anemia, may affect both school performance and behavior. Routine blood tests for anemia, hemoglobin, or hematocrit do not identify this second category.
3. *Iron deficiency with anemia* occurs when the body becomes even further depleted of iron. This group is easy to identify because their hemoglobin or hematocrit levels are low.

Besides the brain, iron deficiency can affect many other systems in the body, such as the gastrointestinal tract, skin, nails, and even the immunologic defense mechanisms. Studies in both animals and in humans have shown that iron deficiency can cause easy fatigability and loss of stamina.

When should parents suspect iron deficiency in their children? The following is a list of some major signs and symptoms that have been shown to be associated with iron deficiency:

1. *Loss of appetite*: This may represent an actual refusal to eat solids or it may be secondary to drinking too much milk.

2. *Failure to thrive*: Some infants with iron deficiency have been reported to have a delay in growth and weight gain.

3. *Increased irritability*: Iron-deficient infants are often more irritable and show a general lack of interest in their surroundings.

4. *Pica*: Pica refers to an infant's craving for eating nonfood substances. Some people believe that there is an association between pica and iron deficiency, but this relationship has never been proven.

5. *Breath-holding*: There is a possible relationship (again unproven) between breath-holding episodes and iron deficiency. If your baby is a breath-holder, it would be advisable to ask your doctor to check for iron deficiency. Although it is true that breath-holding episodes are generally harmless, they can be very frightening to parents.

6. *Easy fatigability*: Getting tired too easily may indicate low iron stores.

7. *Poor school performance*: A number of studies have demonstrated that iron deficiency can affect a child's schoolwork.

Of course, any and all of these symptoms can be caused by something other than iron deficiency. Let's not forget that some kids are just naturally less energetic, more difficult to get along with, less curious, and less intellectually capable than others. Nevertheless, the signs that I have just mentioned sometimes do indicate that a young child is not getting the iron he needs. These signs and symptoms disappear within a very short time after iron intake is increased if, in fact, they were due to iron deficiency.

In a study conducted by Doctors Oski and Honig, eight of twelve iron-deficient children between nine and twenty-six months of age who were given iron by injection for only one week showed a significant increase of ten points or more on the Mental Development Index of the Bayley Scale of Infant Development. In the same study four of eight toddlers who initially scored poorly on the Infant Behavior Record increased their scores one week after being treated with iron, whereas none of the eleven poor-scoring infants in the control group improved. Although iron in injectable form was used in this particular study, other studies with somewhat older children, in which the iron was given orally, produced equally convincing results.

In another recent investigation conducted by Dr. S. Seshadri, a group of anemic five- and six-year-old boys were given supplemental iron for sixty days. A matched control group did not receive any additional iron. Before the study began, both groups were given 12 tests. At the end of two months the boys who had received iron had significantly higher verbal IQs and performance IQ scores, whereas the control group showed no statistically significant changes in their IQ scores.

In my practice I have seen how quickly some children perk up mentally and become easier to get along with when they get enough iron in their diets or via an iron supplement.

Why is too little iron a problem for so many children? The answer is twofold. The first part is simple: Iron-rich foods such as leafy green vegetables and liver appear too infrequently on many dinner tables across the land. But even in homes where these foods are served often, the child in residence may balk at eating them, either because he doesn't like them or—and here it gets more complicated—because he is not hungry enough to eat much of anything. This is the second reason for iron deficiency. Many children still drink enormous quantities of milk each day, much more than they actually need. Milk is filling and an excellent source of calcium but it contains no iron. Too much milk at mealtime can fill up your child just enough to kill his appetite for any other iron-rich foods.

I urge all parents to limit the amount of milk their children drink to no more than three 8-ounce glasses per day. If your youngster drinks two 8-ounce glasses of milk a day, plus a little cheese and some yogurt, he will be getting more than enough of the calcium he needs for good health and development. By cutting milk consumption down a bit your child will probably take a greater interest in eating a wider variety of foods, some of which will contain iron. Fruit juices and sweetened fruit drinks, like milk, can also dull young appetites when drunk at mealtime or just before. Naturally, if you suspect that too much juice is spoiling your child's appetite, offer him less, or dilute the juice with water.

"Less milk, less juice, what's the poor child to drink?" one mother asked after I suggested that she ration these two beverages. My answer? Why, plain water, of course! (Here's a tip for you if your child has never been enthusiastic about tap water:

Pour water into a large plastic bottle or pitcher and put it into the refrigerator to chill. For some reason, unknown to me, water seems more special to a child when it comes from a container instead of the faucet.)

Because we now understand that iron deficiency, even before the anemia develops, can cause significant problems, the only sensible approach is to *prevent* it from ever developing. Even if your infant or child does not have any of the usual signs and symptoms of iron deficiency, you should learn the food sources that are rich in iron and how best to supply adequate daily amounts to your child. Depending on your child's age, from 10 to 18 milligrams of iron per day are needed to prevent iron deficiency. Some key sources of iron are liver (calf, beef, and chicken) and red meats. Other excellent sources of iron are dried fruits, dark-green leafy vegetables, and iron-fortified cereals.

IRON-RICH FOODS

	Quantity	Iron (mg)
Calves liver	3 oz.	9
Lean steak	3 oz.	4.5
Pork chop	3 oz.	4.5
Lamb	3 oz.	3
Turkey, dark meat	3 oz.	2.5
Chicken, dark meat	3 oz.	2
Tuna	3 oz.	2
Dried apricots	1 cup	6
Prune juice	½ cup	1.5
Prunes	½ cup	2
Dates	9	1
Baked beans	½ cup	3
Kidney beans	½ cup	3
Molasses, blackstrap	1 Tb.	3
Raisins	½ cup	2
Tofu	½ cup	2
Fortified cereals:		
Bran buds	½ cup	6

IRON-RICH FOODS

	Quantity	Iron (mg)
Bran Chex	½ cup	4
C. W. Post with Raisins	½ cup	8
Corn Bran	½ cup	6
Fortified Oat Flakes	½ cup	4
40% and 100% Bran Flakes	½ cup	4–6
Golden Grahams	½ cup	3
Life	½ cup	6
Most	½ cup	16
Product 19	½ cup	11
Total	½ cup	11
Wheat germ, toasted	½ cup	5
Cream of Wheat, cooked	½ cup	5
Maypo, cooked	½ cup	4

Not all iron sources are equally absorbed. The iron from animal sources, called heme iron, provides the richest source of iron. The body absorbs less of the iron supplied from plant foods (nonheme iron) such as found in dried fruits, nuts, and leafy green vegetables. Vitamin C enhances the absorption of nonheme iron and so it is especially important to add vitamin C to the meals containing the more poorly absorbed nonheme iron foods. For example, a glass of orange juice with an iron-enriched breakfast cereal increases the absorption of the iron by 250 percent. A slice of cantaloupe with a cup of split pea soup or an orange with a peanut butter sandwich will greatly enhance the iron intake of the meal. The Eden diet includes attractive and delicious food choices and combinations that will supply your child with sufficient iron for optimal health and peak performance.

A colleague of mine called me in consultation to examine a thirteen-year-old boy who was having behavior problems in school. As part of my investigation into this young fellow's difficulties I asked him to keep a one-day food diary. This is what he mailed me:

BREAKFAST	1 oz. sugar-coated cereal (frosted-flakes type)
	½ cup milk
	Orange drink—sweetened
LUNCH	2 slices white bread
	Peanut butter (3 Tbs). and jelly (2 Tbs.)
	2 chocolate chip Cookies
	1 cup grape juice
AFTERNOON SNACK	1 pkg. potato chips
	12 oz. cola
DINNER	¼ lb. french fries
	Fried chicken—thigh and leg
	2 rolls with butter
	¾ cup cole slaw
	12 oz. chocolate milkshake
BEDTIME SNACK	½ pint ice cream

It was obvious from this diary that this young man was being truthful with me. In my experience, food diaries are often inaccurate and omit many between-meal so-called junk food snacks. It also was very clear that he was eating a diet too high in calories, refined sugar and fat, and too low in iron, calcium, vitamin C, and fiber. A blood test showed that he was markedly iron deficient. We corrected his iron deficiency by prescribing a daily iron supplement and putting him on the Eden diet. His school performance and behavior improved dramatically after only three weeks. We didn't know whether this success was due to his new diet or the correction of his iron deficiency, but we didn't much care.

If you suspect that your child has been eating a diet that is low in iron, there is a very good chance that he is iron deficient, with or without anemia. If this is the case, I would suggest that you discuss it with your child's physician. If your child turns out to be iron deficient, it is very easy for your doctor to supplement his diet with a concentrated iron preparation (either in liquid or solid form) and correct the deficiency. Iron is also incorporated in various multivitamin preparations, both in liquid and solid form (iron-fortified vitamins). After that, monitoring your child's daily diet to make certain that he is getting enough iron is essential to prevent it from developing again.

CHAPTER 6
Add More Fiber

Grandma used to call it roughage. She insisted that roughage was important because it helped digest foods and prevented constipation. We now call it fiber, but it is the same old stuff. Grandma was right—fiber does aid in the digestive processes. But now we know that it does much more than that.

Fiber is a varied group of plant residues. Many of these plant residues, found in fruits, vegetables, and whole grains, are not broken down by the digestive enzymes of the gastrointestinal tract and so are not digestible. Even though it is not an actual nutrient, it turns out that fiber is an important component of the diet.

A diet rich in fiber helps protect against a number of gastrointestinal diseases, including appendicitis, diverticulitis, and cancer of the colon and rectum. These gastrointestinal diseases are seen more frequently in our Western civilization where the diet we eat is relatively low in fiber. In societies and cultures whose diets are high in fiber, the incidence of these illnesses is much lower. We don't know for certain why this is so. One reasonable explanation is that fiber helps food pass more quickly through the gastrointestinal tract, and therefore allows less time for the intestine to be in contact with cancer-promoting components of digested food. Doctor Marvin Schneiderman, formerly of the National Cancer Institute, believes that the majority of deaths per year from cancer of the colon and rectum could be prevented by a moderate substitute of high-fiber foods for foods high in saturated fat. Fiber is also important in the prevention and treatment of mild constipation in children. A diet containing whole-grain breads and cereals, fruits and vegetables, together with plenty of fluids helps maintain healthy bowel function. There is recent evidence suggesting that a high fiber diet is also associated with a lower incidence of cardiovascular disease, because such a diet is usually lower in total animal or saturated fat. Further, a diet high in fiber tends to be low in calories and so it is ideal as a natural method of weight control.

Most children now eat diets that are too low in fiber. One reason for this is that food processing removes most of the indigestible fiber from the carbohydrate foods that constitute the major part of the diet. We also tend to choose foods that are low in fiber, such as potato chips instead of potatoes, white bread instead of whole-grain bread, apple juice instead of the fruit itself. Our kids should be encouraged to eat more fruit and vegetables. Besides containing fiber, dark-green, orange, and yellow vegetables such as broccoli, carrots, and sweet potato are rich in beta-carotene, the chemical that the body converts to vitamin A, which is believed to help protect against certain forms of cancer. Fruits and vegetables also contain vitamin C and folic acid, important nutrients for disease prevention. In animal studies, cancers have also been inhibited by some vegetables found in the cabbage family, such as broccoli, Brussels sprouts, cauliflower, and cabbage.

The soluble fiber found in fruits and in vegetables, oats, rye, barley, and legumes has also been found to be helpful in lowering the level of blood sugar. This is particularly important for people with high blood sugar, such as diabetics.

To increase your child's fiber intake, the following foods are recommended in the Eden diet:

Breads made from:	Whole-wheat, pumpernickel, and rye flours
Whole-grain dry cereals:	Bran cereals, puffed wheat, shredded wheat, Grape-Nuts, Wheaties,

	Corn Chex, Bran Flakes, Total, and Post Toasties
Cooked cereals and grains:	Oatmeal, Ralston, Wheatena, kasha (buckwheat groats), barley, brown rice
Other whole grains:	Unprocessed or raw bran, corn bran, whole-wheat pasta
Vegetables:	Peas, spinach, corn, broccoli, potatoes with skins, yams with skins, eggplant, carrots, Brussels sprouts, green beans, cabbage, and beets
Legumes (dried beans and peas):	Lentils, black beans, chick peas, kidney beans, lima beans, black-eyed peas
Fruits:	*Dried:* Figs, prunes, apricots, dates, raisins *Fresh:* (with skin) Apples, pears, bananas, peaches, tangerines, apricots, plums, nectarines, oranges, cantaloupe, honeydew, watermelon *Berries:* Raspberries, blackberries, cranberries and strawberries
Snacks:	Popcorn, rye crackers, whole-wheat crackers, graham crackers, Cheerios

To help you increase the fiber in your family's diet:

1. Serve whole-wheat, pumpernickel, or oatmeal bread instead of white bread.
2. Serve bran cereal and oatmeal.
3. Serve fresh fruits and vegetables often (with skins).
4. Top dishes with nuts, seeds, or berries.
5. Serve salads every day.
6. Eat fresh fruit, raw vegetables, and rye or whole-wheat crackers as snacks.

These foods will supply your child with enough fiber for optimal nutritional health and reduced risk of disease. And if he grows accustomed to high-fiber foods now, he'll begin to develop a taste for fruits, vegetables, and whole grains that will more than likely carry over as he grows up and becomes an adult.

CHAPTER 7
Fight the S.O.B. Syndrome

Overcrowding, increasing automobile traffic, less open space, and fewer play areas, all contribute to reducing opportunities for kids to run around and play. Add to that television, home computers, and video games—all making it very easy for a child to become sedentary and physically inactive. The result of all this is what I call the S.O.B. syndrome—the "*S*itting *O*n *B*ehind" syndrome. It really should be called the S.O.A. syndrome but somehow that doesn't have the same ring to it as S.O.B. Television watching is still the major culprit in creating this condition. Children spend hundreds upon hundreds of hours sitting in front of TV sets, their only real exercise an occasional trip to the bathroom or to the refrigerator to stock up on another supply of junk food snacks.

This lack of exercise in childhood is widespread. A recent large-scale U.S. government survey proves this. The Department of Health and Human Services studied 3800 school-aged children from grades 5 through 12 in nineteen states. Their conclusions were as follows:

1. One half of these children did not exercise enough to develop healthy hearts and lungs (less than 20 minutes per day three times a week).
2. Only 36 percent of these children took physical education classes each day in school.

3. This group was found to be fatter than a similar group of children examined back in the 1960s.

A review of a recent survey of the President's Council on Physical Fitness dealing with adults also proves the lack of sufficient exercise in children. This study showed that very few of the large group of nonexercising adults exercised very much when they were children. Almost one-half of all the adults in the United States don't participate in any specific physical activity for the purpose of exercise. Only 35 percent of grownups regularly engage in any type of vigorous physical exercise. Most significant of all was the fact that two-thirds of the nonexercising adults actually believed that they were getting sufficient exercise. There is little question that this large group of sedentary adults was started on the road to their inactivity during childhood, when proper exercise habits were not instilled and cultivated. The purpose of the Eden Fitness Program is to change all that.

Achieving physical fitness through regular exercise must be a way of life with every single child. Exercise must be incorporated into the daily routine of all children. You must do everything possible to encourage your child's physical activity, and the earlier you start the better.

YOUR EXAMPLE

Children learn by example. This is an important axiom that you should always remember. To illustrate, if you don't want your child to become a smoker, stop smoking yourself. Statistics show much higher incidence of smoking among children raised in homes where the parents smoke than in nonsmoking households. If you want your child to grow up physically fit, as I'm sure you do, lead the way yourself. An exercise and fitness program that is geared to tone up your muscles and get rid of your extra fat will set the example your child needs. A family that exercises together not only stays together, but has a wonderful time along the way.

There are many satisfactions and health benefits that derive from regular vigorous exercise and sports programs in childhood. The most significant benefit is that the child will be more likely to continue to exercise more regularly as an adult. The health implications for the adult are obvious. Regular exercise helps prevent obesity, high blood pressure, strokes, and heart attacks. It is the key to improving cardiovascular health and increases both the quality and the length of life.

Those of us who exercise regularly have always been aware of the "high" or feeling of well-being associated with it. Recently, we have learned why this natural "high" develops. There are naturally-occurring substances in the body, opiumlike compounds called betaendorphins that produce pain-free states. Studies have shown that extended vigorous exercise raises the blood level of these endorphins and this explains the feeling of well-being. Exercise also relieves tendencies toward depression and so promotes an attitude of optimism and positive self-esteem. This is true for children as well.

Regular exercise (especially aerobic exercise) reduces the risk of an adult suffering a heart attack. It keeps all the muscles of the body (including the heart muscles) in tone, and this is an important safeguard. Exercise also develops a collateral coronary circulation and this is yet another protection against a heart attack. Of extreme importance is the fact that exercise has been shown to lower the total blood cholesterol level and this further lowers the risk of heart trouble. Probably of greatest significance in terms of its relationship to heart attacks is the fact that exercise raises the level of the high-density lipoproteins in the blood. High-density lipoproteins (H.D.L.s) are associated with a significantly reduced risk of coronary heart disease. These H.D.L.s appear to remove cholesterol molecules from the coronary artery walls. Finally, exercise also lowers the level of the low-density lipoproteins (L.D.L.s) that have been clearly implicated in the process of atherosclerosis. L.D.L.s seem to be responsible for depositing cholesterol crystals on to the artery walls (see pages 000). For all these reasons it is clear that a regular exercise program is excellent protection against heart attacks. Please remember that if your child does not learn to enjoy strenuous physical activity now, it will be much less likely that he will do any better as an adult. A sedentary lifestyle then will increase his risk of heart attack.

LOWER BLOOD PRESSURE

Another important health advantage of regular vigorous exercise is related to blood pressure. It works two ways. First, regular exercise burns up calories, and weight reduction has been shown to lower blood pressure. Second, exercise programs have been shown to lower blood pressure even without accompanying weight loss. Doctor D. Goldring and associates conducted a study on a group of adolescents with persistent hypertension. They were put on a structured exercise training program three times a week for six months. The result was a significant lowering of blood pressure. The great majority of the adolescents in this study were found to be unenthusiastic about exercising and preferred more sedentary activities. This raises the possibility that a physically inactive lifestyle may predispose a susceptible child to high blood pressure. Because high blood pressure can cause a stroke, anybody who doesn't exercise regularly is just looking for trouble.

AEROBIC BENEFITS

Aerobic or endurance exercises are best because these types of exercise speed up metabolism and also improve lung and heart function. Aerobic exercises result in the lungs being able to move more air in and out with each breath. These exercises also train the heart to pump more and more blood through the lungs and into the working muscles each minute. The strongest hearts are the ones that can pump the most oxygen-rich blood per unit time. This increased oxygen uptake—the amount of oxygen that the body is able to extract from inhaled air and transport to muscles—is considered by exercise physiologists to be the ultimate measure of physical fitness.

Among aerobic exercises are the following:

Brisk walking
Jogging
Running
Cycling
Skating
Lap swimming
Rope jumping
Aerobic dancing

The effects of aerobic training are as follows:

1. Lowers heart rate, makes the heart more efficient, and develops a stronger pump action.
2. Lowers blood pressure.
3. Allows lungs to hold more air and breathe more slowly.

Whenever possible, encourage your child to become involved in one or another of these aerobic exercises. If he learns to enjoy this type of exercise, he stands a good chance of maintaining this habit as he grows up. For the adult, aerobic exercises are crucial to maintain maximum cardiovascular health. At the core of the Eden Fitness Program are aerobic activities.

CARRY-OVER SPORTS

Besides aerobic exercises it is important to encourage children to learn "carry-over" sports. Carry-over sports refer to those activities that can be continued throughout life. While baseball, basketball and football are excellent sports, it is pretty difficult to organize two teams and a game after graduating from school. Therefore, sports that don't require large numbers of people or even anyone else, are the ones that are easier to continue to play as an adult. Some examples of carry-over sports are: bicycling, swimming, jogging, skating (all aerobic) and tennis and other racquet games. The earlier your child learns the skills appropriate to the "carry-over" sport, the more likely he will excel in the activity and so he'll have more fun doing it.

Boys and girls are similar in size and physique until around age ten when girls begin their pubertal growth spurt. Therefore, it is perfectly reasonable for boys and girls to compete until then and play on the same teams.

Children of small or slight stature should be encouraged in sports activities such as tennis, swimming, soccer and track rather than in the collision sports, football, ice-hockey and lacrosse, where they will be at a marked disadvantage.

Between ages ten and fourteen collision sports are inappropriate. Participating in such activities at that age risks serious bone and joint injury.

PART II

DIET-PLAN MENUS FOR HEALTHIER EATING

CHAPTER 8
General Guidelines and Cooking Tips

The Eden diet plan is based on medically sound dietary recommendations, with a particular emphasis on pleasing the palates of children. The diet has been developed with the following goals in mind:

1. To maintain the ideal body weight for your child by supplying sufficient calories for optimal growth and development.
2. To avoid obesity by providing the correct number of calories for your child's age and body weight, by supplying separate menu plans for normal and overweight children.
3. To decrease your child's risk of developing heart attack, stroke, high blood pressure, and cancer of the colon and breast later on in life by introducing a diet lower in fat, cholesterol, and salt.
4. To decrease the discomfort of constipation as well as the risk of diverticulitis, diverticulosis, and colon cancer as an adult by encouraging the consumption of foods high in dietary fiber.
5. To decrease the risk of developing iron deficiency with its potential of causing learning disabilities, easy fatigability, and irritability.
6. To decrease the risk of other potentially avoidable diseases, such as adult onset diabetes and osteoporosis.
7. To change your family's dietary habits for the better.

DIET-PLAN MENUS FOR HEALTHIER EATING

Specific Guidelines:

Calories: The number of calories will vary according to the recommended caloric intake for children in each age group. Overweight children will be given slightly fewer calories—200 calories per day less in the younger age groups, 300 calories per day less in the older age groups.

			Average	*Overweight*
Toddler	(1–3 yrs.)		1300	1100
Preschool	(3–5 yrs.)		1700	1500
School age	(6–10 yrs.)		2400	2100
Teens	(10–15 yrs.)	male	2700	2400
		female	2100	1800
	(15–18 yrs.)	male	2200	2000
		female	1900	1600

Fats: Fats will be kept to 30 percent of total calorie intake or less, and saturated fats will be reduced to about one third of total fats.

Cholesterol: Cholesterol intake will be kept down to less than 300 milligrams per day.

Vitamins and minerals: The menus supply at least two-thirds of the RDA for all vitamins and minerals. In particular, the adequate intake of vitamin C, iron, and calcium will be stressed.

Sugar: Little refined sugar is used. The use of fruits and fruit juices is encouraged.

Fiber: Dietary fiber is in the range of 10–20 grams per day, a moderately high intake.

Salt: Salt use will be minimized.

To accomplish these specific guidelines, the Eden diet recommends:

1. Sufficient calories for adequate growth and development.
2. More fish and skinless chicken and turkey to reach and stay at ideal body weight. Limit beef, pork, and lamb. Avoid fatty meats such as bacon and sausages.

3. Preparing fish, chicken, and turkey by broiling, baking, steaming, or poaching. These methods of cooking do not require the addition of fat or oil. Limit or avoid all deep-fried foods.
4. Limiting the intake of egg yolks in cooking, baking, or for general consumption to no more than 3–4 egg yolks per week. (Egg yolks are the highest, most concentrated source of cholesterol commonly eaten in this country.)
5. Switching from whole milk and whole milk products to low-fat and skimmed milk products. Avoid the frequent use of high-fat foods such as ice cream, whipped cream, and some cheeses.
6. Serving salads, fresh and frozen vegetables, raw and cooked fruits often, as snacks, as a component of meals and for desserts.
7. Eating whole-wheat bread and cereal, brown rice, pumpernickel and dark rye breads, and other whole-grain products.
8. Using more recipes containing dried peas and beans, such as navy bean, lentil, and split pea soups, chili, hummus, and bean dips.
9. Limiting the use of highly sugared products, and those foods that contain artificial colorings, nitrates, and nitrites.
10. Limiting salt intake by:

    (a) Using little or no salt during cooking.
    (b) Keeping the salt shaker off the table at mealtimes.
    (c) Seasoning foods with herbs, spices, lemon juice, and pepper, rather than with salt.
    (d) Choosing fresh or frozen vegetables in place of canned because a great deal of salt is added during the canning process.
    (e) Serving few or no foods with high-salt content. (If salt or sodium or a substance having sodium as part of its name such as sodium citrate is among the few ingredients listed on the label, you can be sure it's a high-salt content.)

MENU BASICS

The following are the principles behind seven days of menus of the Eden diet. If you prefer not to follow the specific meal plans, simply refer to these guidelines.

BREAKFAST	Fruit or fruit juice, unsweetened whole-grain cereal or bread Low-fat or skim milk or yogurt
LUNCH	Pasta or whole-grain bread Low-fat meat, fish, and poultry Salad or cut-up vegetables with low-fat dressing or spread Low-fat or skim milk
DINNER	Pasta, rice, or whole-grain bread Low-fat meat, fish, or poultry Salad or cut-up vegetables Low-fat or skim-milk product
SNACK	Piece of fruit or unsweetened fruit juice or Whole-grain crackers or cookie or Raw vegetables with low-fat dip or Low-fat yogurt

Time snacks according to your child's needs. The times indicated in the menus are only suggestions.

HEALTHIER COOKERY

The Eden diet plans are not only recommended for children of all ages but for the whole family as well. For healthier cookery for all, we suggest that you modify your favorite recipes according to the following eight principles:

1. Avoid recipes that call for deep frying. These recipes always contain large amounts of fat.
2. When sautéing or stir-frying meats or vegetables, try to use half the amount of oil or butter called for in the recipe. You probably won't miss the extra fat and you can save 120 calories for every tablespoon of fat avoided.
3. Use a nonstick skillet to avoid the use of fat in cooking. Use a nonstick spray for muffin pans and cookie sheets.
4. When thickening a white sauce, try mixing the flour with the cold liquid instead of combining flour with butter, and simmer for 5 minutes over low heat. Add 2 tablespoons of Parmesan cheese for a low-fat cheese sauce.
5. When following recipes on a box, the same practice holds: Instead of adding 4 tablespoons of butter or margarine to a powdered cheese mixture that is added to macaroni, try adding 1–2 teaspoons. Your child will not notice the difference.
6. When cooking spaghetti, macaroni, or rice, avoid salting the water. Your child will not miss the extra sodium.
7. Use fewer egg yolks in cooking. For an omelette or scrambled eggs, try using an egg white with one whole egg instead of two whole eggs to decrease the fat and cholesterol content. Many recipes for cakes can also benefit from this substitution.
8. Use low-fat salad dressings instead of those based on oil, mayonnaise, or sour cream. Low-fat dressing bases can be made from low-fat buttermilk, blended cottage cheese, or yogurt. Add garlic, vinegar, lemon juice, herbs, and spices to taste.

MILK, CHEESE, BUTTER, OIL

EAT MORE OF THESE*
Nonfat fortified milk; skim milk; low-fat yogurt; buttermilk (made with skim milk); low-fat cottage cheese; cheeses containing less than 5 percent butterfat; margarine (soft tub or

*Reproduced with the permission of Wyeth Laboratories. © 1984, Wyeth Laboratories.

stick made with corn, cottonseed, soy, safflower or sunflower oils *only*); corn oil; sunflower oil; safflower oil; peanut oil; soy oil

EAT MODERATE AMOUNTS OF THESE*
1 percent or 2 percent fat-fortified milk; frozen yogurt; low-fat, hard cheese; ice milk; soft margarine; mayonnaise; skimmed, evaporated milk (good for cooking in place of cream or whole milk)

EAT LESS OF THESE*
Whole and chocolate milk; canned, evaporated whole milk; buttermilk; whole cream; hard and cream cheeses; sour cream; high-fat ice cream; butter; shortening; lard; bacon fat; eggs

MEAT, FISH, POULTRY

EAT MORE OF THESE
Fresh or fresh-frozen fish; tuna; crab; scallops; chicken; turkey; cornish hen (without the skin); lean veal

EAT MODERATE AMOUNTS OF THESE
(Trim off fat) Flank steak; beef filet; leg of lamb; sirloin; pork (whole rump, center shank); ham (center slices); rib eye; ground beef; pork loin; boiled ham; chicken frankfurter

EAT LESS OF THESE
(Trim off fat) Corned beef (brisket); hamburger (commercial); steaks (club and rib); rib roast; breast of lamb; spareribs; ground pork; deviled ham; breast of veal; regular frankfurter; cold cuts; fried chicken (with skin or prepared with saturated oil); duck and goose; sausage and bacon; liver, heart, and other organ meats; sardines

---

*Reproduced with the permission of Wyeth Laboratories. © 1984, Wyeth Laboratories.

VEGETABLES

EAT MORE OF THESE
(Fresh is best, raw or steamed) Asparagus; bean sprouts; beets; broccoli; Brussels sprouts; cauliflower; cabbage; carrots; eggplant; green beans; string beans; squash (summer); zucchini; cucumbers; watercress; lettuce; corn; peas

EAT MODERATE AMOUNTS OF THESE
Canned vegetables (some are high in salt, check label); frozen vegetables (without added salt); canned vegetable soups (read label for salt content); stir-fried vegetables prepared in small amount of polyunsaturated fat

EAT LESS OF THESE
Vegetables fried in butter or other saturated fats; frozen vegetables (processed with salt, such as mixed vegetables); vegetables made with cream and butter sauces

FRUITS, FRUIT JUICES

EAT MORE OF THESE
Apples/apple juice; apricots (fresh or dried); bananas; berries; cherries; dates; figs; grapes; oranges; peaches; plums; grapefruit; raisins; prunes; fresh fruit juices without added sugar

EAT MODERATE AMOUNTS OF THESE
Fruits canned in juices; fruits canned in water; fruit ice

EAT LESS OF THESE
Fruits canned in heavy syrup; fruit drinks; glazed fruit (all fruits to which sodium, coloring or sodium benzoate has been added)

STARCHES, CEREALS, GRAINS

EAT MORE OF THESE
Whole-wheat, rye, pumpernickel, raisin breads; cornmeal; whole-wheat pasta; brown rice; potatoes (sweet or white); yams; pumpkin; beans and lentils; grits; wheat germ; oatmeal; puffed rice

EAT MODERATE AMOUNTS OF THESE
White bread; refined pasta; white rice; refined, unsweetened cereal; low-salt, whole-wheat crackers made with soybean oil

EAT LESS OF THESE
Instant potatoes; other prepared potato products (these are high in salt); french fries; commercially prepared foods such as macaroni and cheese, lasagna, pizza, cheese blintzes (homemade foods are better); sweetened cereal; sweet rolls; salted crackers made with palm and/or coconut oil

SNACKS, DESSERTS, NUTS

EAT MORE OF THESE
Fresh fruits and vegetables; dried fruits (raisins); low-fat yogurt; popcorn (unsalted, unbuttered); homemade oatmeal cookies (made with safflower, cottonseed, or corn oil, raisins and raw apples)

EAT MODERATE AMOUNTS OF THESE
Low-fat or part-skim cheeses; ice milk; peanut butter; unsalted peanuts; walnuts; almonds; pecans (fat content is mainly monounsaturated)

EAT LESS OF THESE
Commercial cakes; cookies; pies; candy; ice cream; potato and corn chips; salted peanuts; pretzels

DRESSINGS, SAUCES, CONDIMENTS

EAT MORE OF THESE
Natural herbs and spices; fresh onion; garlic powder; pepper; lemon juice; tomato; lettuce; onion; cucumber

EAT MODERATE AMOUNTS OF THESE
Unsalted, low-fat salad dressing; homemade dressing made with polyunsaturated oils (safflower, corn, or cottonseed)

EAT LESS OF THESE
All are high in sodium: steak sauces; soy sauce; salt; garlic, celery and onion salts; meat tenderizers; celery seed; horseradish; commercial salad dressings; salted meat gravy; chili sauce; butter sauces

CHAPTER 9

Feeding Your Infant

Proper nutrition during the first year of life is very important to the future health of your child. Despite current knowledge about what is considered optimal nutrition, it is all too easy to make mistakes.

The faulty infant feeding practices that are so prevalent nowadays often lead to obesity, iron deficiency, and increased strain on the kidneys. Among the major mistakes during the first twelve months of life are switching to regular cow's milk too soon, starting solid foods too early, encouraging too much sugar and salt, and overfeeding.

BABY'S FIRST FOOD

The best way to feed an infant during the first year is to breast feed. Human milk has been proven to be ideally suited to all the infant's nutritional needs. What's more, there is strong evidence that breast milk contains certain antibodies that protect the baby against many viral and bacterial infections, especially those involving the gastrointestinal tract. We also have some preliminary data that support the theory that breast-fed babies may be better able to handle cholesterol later on in life than those who are bottle-fed. Breast feeding is easy, economical, hygienic, and ideal from the psychological and emotional points of view. I would encourage all expectant mothers to consider its many advantages.

The sensible time to decide whether or not to breast feed is during the pregnancy and not after the infant is born. The 1970s witnessed an increased interest in breast feeding. Compared to the 1950s, twice as many new mothers chose to breast feed. Now in the 1980s, I am happy to report that even more women are choosing to breast feed. There is still a large dropout rate, however, so that after three months almost half the breast-feeding mothers have stopped.

When breast feeding is unsuccessful, inappropriate because of lifestyle, stopped before the infant is one year of age, or simply if the mother decides against it, there is no reason for her to feel guilty. There is a rational and sensible alternative for those women, namely, the commercially available formulas. Although not identical to breast milk, they come very close in their nutrient mix. For the bottle-fed infant, the Committee on Nutrition of the American Academy of Pediatrics recommends the use of an iron-fortified formula to prevent iron deficiency. I agree.

Whichever way you feed your baby, it is important not to overfeed. If you can manage to avoid overfeeding from the very beginning, there is a good chance of sparing your child all the disadvantages and potential health hazards of growing up fat. How can an infant be overfed? One sure way is never to allow your baby to decide when the feeding is over. I see this happening more often among bottle-feeding mothers than among the breast-feeding group. The bottle-feeding mother knows exactly how many ounces of formula there were to start with, and she will see to it that every last drop goes down the baby's throat. On the other hand, breasts are not marked off in ounces. The breast-feeding mother has no way of knowing how many ounces her baby has consumed and so the feeding usually stops when the baby appears satiated rather than when the mother thinks the feeding should be over.

Crying also may lead to overfeeding. Many new parents automatically assume that every time their baby cries she is hungry, but this just is not so. Infants cry for many other reasons besides being hungry. They cry when they are lonely, thirsty for water, bored, or gassy. Keeping in mind that it takes at least three hours for an infant's stomach to empty after an adequate feeding, it is unlikely that she's crying from hunger if the screaming starts one hour after the feeding. With these facts in mind it usually isn't difficult for new parents to learn to differentiate the different types of crying.

Whether you breast feed or use a commercial formula, it is important *not* to switch to regular cow's milk too soon. This milk may be ideal for calves, but it was not designed for human babies. It contains much more salt and protein than either breast milk or formula. This extra salt and protein uses up a good deal of baby's body water in order to be eliminated from the body, which puts an increased strain on the infant's kidneys. If a baby gets sick (i.e. from diarrhea), dehydration will occur sooner in the infant fed regular milk than in the breast-fed or formula-fed baby. Another danger is that a certain percentage of infants less than one year of age who are fed cow's milk bleed into their gastrointestinal tracts, causing iron deficiency and iron-deficiency anemia. Finally, regular cow's milk contains no iron, and this also leads to iron deficiency.

In my office I encourage mothers to continue to breast feed for as long as possible. If, for whatever reason, breast feeding is stopped before one year of age, I switch the infant to an iron-fortified commercial formula, not to regular cow's milk.

You don't have to stop breast feeding if you go to work full time outside the home. Breast milk can be pumped and stored to be used during the feedings when the mother is away from the house, or, if this is inappropriate or too difficult, supplementary feedings of formula can be given. Infants learn rapidly to accept both the breast and bottle in these situations. Babies who are fed formula from the start should continue for at least nine months and up to one year. After that, regular cow's milk is fine.

FLUORIDE FOR STRONGER TEETH

Besides breast milk or formula, we recommend the use of a multivitamin preparation with or without fluoride, depending on the level of fluoride in the water of the community. There are still some who question the use of fluoride, but its advantages have been proven beyond a shadow of a doubt. As a result of fluoride administration there has been a dramatic decrease in the incidence of dental caries in infants and children. New recommendations regarding fluoride administration were recently published by the Committee on Nutrition of the American Academy of Pediatrics. They recommend that fluoride supplementation start at two weeks of age and continue until age sixteen. If you find out that your local water supply does not contain sufficient fluoride, your infant will require extra fluoride. This can be given either in combination with a multivitamin preparation or in the form of fluoride drops. Both for breast-fed and formula-fed infants the daily dose of fluoride is determined by the level of fluoride in the water supply. I would suggest that you check this out with your baby's physician.

THE RIGHT TIME FOR SOLID FOODS

The age at which solids should be introduced into the infant's diet is important in terms of optimal infant nutrition. The current recommendations of the Committee on Nutrition of the American Academy of Pediatrics is to withhold all solid foods until the infant is at least four months of age. The current consensus among authorities is that solid foods be started somewhere between four and six months of age. I am in agreement, and this is the approach of the Eden diet.

These current recommendations are a drastic change from those of ten or twenty years ago. At that time, it was usual to start some solids when the infant was only three or four weeks old. There are three important reasons for this change in the approach to infant feeding:

1. Although we have no hard statistical data, many experts believe that the added calories provided by solid foods before four months of age are unnecessary from the nutritional point of view and probably contribute to excessive weight gain.
2. There is some presumptive evidence that the too-early introduction of solid foods can cause food allergies and perhaps even respiratory allergies such as bronchial asthma later in life.
3. As Dr. Samuel Fomon, a leading authority on infant nutrition has pointed out, a baby less than four or five months old has little or no control over her head and neck muscles. This means that any baby younger than this who is fed solids is unable to turn away from the feeding when satiated; and so the mother and not the baby decides how much food goes down the throat. The result is overfeeding. By four or five months of age, however, most infants have achieved good control over their head and neck muscles, and so they are able to turn away when satisfied, the signal that the feeding is over.

Many parents are overly anxious to introduce solid foods because they believe that this will help their baby sleep through the night. There is no proof of this, but even if it is true, it isn't a good enough reason to start solids too soon. If the withholding of solids until your baby is four or five months old causes you to get up more often for night feedings, in the long run it is well worth the extra effort.

Despite these current recommendations, a number of studies show that a large percentage of babies are still being fed solid foods much too early. A recent Massachusetts survey of 268 infants less than six months old demonstrated that by two months of age 57 percent were eating cereal and by three months of age the number had increased to 87 percent. The message about delaying the introduction of solid foods is just beginning to have some effect on current feeding practices, but there is still a long way to go. It has been my experience that breast-feeding mothers are usually less anxious to start their infants on solid foods than the bottle-feeding mothers.

BRINGING SOLIDS INTO YOUR BABY'S DIET

The schedule for the introduction of solid foods should be individualized because some babies have larger appetites than others. An infant who drinks more than one quart of formula each day, and continually cries for more between feedings, obviously need solids sooner than a baby who drinks less but is content between feedings. The following chart outlines the average schedule of the Eden diet for the introduction of solids.

Age in months	Type of food	Time
4–5	Precooked baby cereals,* twice a day	Morning and evening
5–6	Strained single fruits†, twice a day	Morning and evening
6–7	Strained vegetables†	Lunch
7–8	Strained meats	Lunch
	Plain yogurt	Snack
	Baby juices, no sugar added	Between meals
8–9	Egg yolk—strained, commercial, or home-cooked	Morning (every other day)
10–12	Cottage cheese, toast, teething biscuits, pieces of banana, and other finger foods	

*Cereals are mixed with formula.
†Fruits and vegetables are fed without formula.

You will note in the chart that I suggest giving egg yolk only every other day. There is a reason for this. Eggs are certainly an excellent food from the nutritional point of view, but egg yolk is very rich in cholesterol. Because of this, the Eden diet contains no more than three to four eggs per week throughout childhood and beyond. Because eating habits and patterns are established early in life, starting your infant on eggs every other day makes very good sense to me.

Let me caution you about "nursing bottle" caries. Babies who suck on a bottle of juice or milk while lying down for extended periods of time destroy their teeth. The important point to remember is that your baby should always drink juice or formula in an upright position. If your baby must have a bottle in order to fall asleep, give her water, with no sugar added.

Foods should be introduced one at a time so that if the infant reacts adversely, the particular offending food can be identified and eliminated. Start by giving the baby one teaspoon the first day and gradually increasing the amount each day. It is good practice to wait three to four days before adding the next food to make certain that the baby does not develop an intolerance, such as diarrhea, vomiting, or rash.

Infant cereal is usually the first food to be introduced into the baby's diet. They are all fortified with iron, in a form that is easily and readily digested and absorbed. At about four to five months of age, breast-fed babies and infants on formulas that are not iron fortified need additional iron. By this age most infants have depleted almost all the iron they received from their mothers during pregnancy.

A NOTE ON SALT AND SUGAR

The sequence of the solid foods to be added to the baby's diet is not important. What is important is *not* to add sugar or salt to a baby's food. The baby food manufacturers have removed added salt from all their products and added sugar from most of them. The amount of salt and sugar that is naturally occurring is more than adequate for the baby's nutritional needs. We advise parents *not* to season their baby's foods based on their own food preferences. This also applies to the foods you prepare yourself for the baby. No baby is born craving extra salt. Any baby offered drinks or foods with added sugar very soon becomes addicted to the extra sugar and will continue to demand sugar-laden foods as she grows older.

I would like especially to caution against using honey during the first year of life. Studies have shown that honey may be associated with a very serious disease called botulism in infants up to one year of age, especially those less than six months old. The U.S. Center for Disease Control and the Honey Industry Council of America Inc. both agree that there is no place for honey during an infant's first twelve months of life.

BALANCE IT RIGHT!

It is interesting to note that during the first year infants are usually fed lots of fruits and vegetables, which is a good thing. Not only are fruits and vegetables healthy for the infant, but they are just as healthy for the growing child because they are full of so many important vitamins and high in fiber. But what often happens around one year of age and during the toddler period (one to three years) is that as children are switched to regular table foods, they are offered less fruits and vegetables because of the way the rest of the family eats. This is a serious, faulty feeding practice that must be stopped. The Eden diet consists of plentiful daily portions of fruits and vegetables— from infancy through adolescence and beyond. Contrary to popular belief, children who are offered a variety of fruits and vegetables enjoy eating them.

Between nine and twelve months of age your baby should be introduced to many different nutritious foods, one by one. At this age she should be served three well-balanced meals each day, containing daily servings from each of the four basic food groups:

1. Meats: Includes meat, poultry, and fish with alternatives of eggs, dried beans, and soybeans. Fatty meats should be avoided and the total number of eggs per week should never exceed three to four.
2. Vegetables and fruits: Includes all fruits and vegetables, in abundance.
3. Milk: Includes formula, cheese, and yogurt.
4. Breads and cereals: Includes breads and cereals that are whole-grained or enriched; also includes rice and pasta.

Many babies are introduced to regular table foods during this period, whereas still others prefer strained or junior foods. In either case, as we have stated earlier, remember not to add extra sugar or salt to your baby's food.

At about nine to twelve months of age many babies suddenly rebel against food. This decrease in appetite is normal and you need not worry about it. Because growth slows at this age, the body requires less food. A baby should never be forced to eat when she's not hungry. Allow your baby to eat as much or as little as she wants rather than as much as you think she needs.

This nine- to twelve-month-old period is notorious for the start of iron deficiency. First of all, at this time many babies are switched to regular cow's milk, which contains practically no iron. They drink a great deal of cow's milk, while at the same time they eat very little solid food. This combination can rapidly lead to iron deficiency and iron deficiency anemia (the entire subject of iron deficiency is discussed in detail in Chapter 5). Because iron deficiency may be associated with learning disabilities later on, it is essential that you prevent it. A nine- to twelve-month-old baby who is drinking regular cow's milk and not iron-fortified formula must be offered infant cereals, green vegetables, meats, and eggs—all good sources of iron. If your baby refuses to eat these foods, supplementary iron should be given, either incorporated in the multivitamin preparation or separately. I suggest that you discuss this with your pediatrician.

FAT AND YOUR INFANT

The facts about obesity in infancy are quite clear: Fat babies have a greater chance of ending up fat adults than do normal-weight or thin babies. If you think that your baby is gaining weight too rapidly, her doctor should be consulted about it.

Just look at the baby. If she looks fat, she is fat. It isn't very difficult to notice rolls of fat and extra chins. One rule of thumb that you might find useful is that on average, a baby doubles her birth weight by five months of age and triples it by age one. For example, if your baby weighed 6 pounds at birth, she should weigh about 12 pounds at five months of age and about 18 pounds at a year. If instead, she already weighs 18 pounds by the time she's six months old, that's too much. Take it up with her doctor the next time she's examined.

If your breast-fed baby is gaining weight too rapidly, there is nothing you can do about it except realize that for some unexplained reason these babies usually slim down without any trouble once breast feeding stops. If your baby is being fed formula and gaining weight too rapidly, I suggest that you ask her doctor about diluting the formula with a little water in order to cut down the calories. This is what I advise in my practice. *Never* use skim milk (which is fat-free) during the first year of life, because it has even more salt and protein in it than regular cow's milk. Besides, infants need the fat for proper growth and development.

If you follow these Eden diet suggestions, your infant will receive a well-balanced and nutritionally sound diet. It rarely is necessary to coax a baby to eat. Mealtime should never become a contest between parent and baby; rather, it should be a relaxed and pleasant time. If your baby refuses to eat, she just isn't hungry. She won't starve if she skips a meal. Her appetite should be the only factor in determining how much food she should eat.

CHAPTER 10
Feeding Your High-Energy Toddler

What a difference just a few short months can make! Since birth your baby has probably tripled his weight and grown 50 percent beyond his original height. His development, from a helpless, relatively immobile infant to a lusty little high-energy explorer who *never* seems to sit still, took less than one year. Whereas at first he had few options with regard to asserting his will, now he's learned dozens of new ways to let you know how he feels about things. In a sense, he's broken through an age barrier: On reaching his first birthday he left infancy behind and entered "toddlerhood," and a toddler he'll be until he is three.

These are challenging years for parents. Not the least among your challenges as a concerned mother or father is to continue to make sure your child gets the proper food and exercise so necessary for optimal health. If your infant was put on the Eden Fitness Program soon after he was born, keep up the good work as he moves into this second stage of his life. If not, now is the time to begin. It certainly is not too late for toddlers (as a matter of fact it isn't too late for you young parents in your twenties or thirties, or even for grandparents in their sixties or beyond). Thus if you discovered this book well after your child has crossed the great divide between infancy and toddlerhood, welcome aboard! By beginning now to instill the correct food and exercise habits in your toddler, you will be laying the groundwork for better health for a lifetime.

TOO MUCH OF THE WRONG FOODS

For most children in the United States today, getting enough food is not the problem. More commonly, difficulties arise because of too much of the wrong foods. A number of factors come into play at about the time your baby reaches his first birthday—factors that often result in his getting too much of the wrong foods. To better understand how these factors work, let's consider what typically happens to the toddler and his parents at this crucial age.

In my experience as a pediatrician, I have found that during the first year, parents are very careful about what they feed their baby. This concern tends to taper off after age one. Part of this may in fact be related to the baby's pediatrician. During the first year of life, parents routinely bring their infant to the doctor for frequent checkups—every one or two months. At each of these visits, the pediatrician gives specific instructions about the types of foods to feed the baby and when to add new ones. But about the time of the baby's first birthday, not only do the regular visits to the pediatrician become less frequent (now every three to six months), but parents are usually told that now it is okay to switch the infant from baby foods to table foods. In other words, the pediatrician no longer monitors the child's diet as closely as before. At the same time, that diet undergoes big changes as the toddler begins to eat basically the same foods as his parents and older siblings.

If the family diet is a healthy one, all is well and good. Unfortunately, the typical American family eats the typical American diet—too high in calories, fat, cholesterol, refined sugar, and salt, and too low in fiber and iron. It's the wrong diet for everybody, but it's just as wrong for the toddler as it is for the older members of his family. It is wrong for the toddler because it gives him more than is good for him of some of the nutrients and, paradoxically, less than he needs of the others.

For the toddler there is practically no risk of developing a heart attack, hypertension, or a nutrition-related cancer. However, the diet you feed your toddler now becomes the diet he'll eat all his life, and that's the trouble. The adorably plump baby can easily become a fat toddler unless the parents take an active role in preventing it. Obesity is not healthy for anyone, including the toddler. Studies have shown that fat toddlers are more likely to catch certain respiratory infections than thin or normal-weight toddlers, and they have also been shown to be more accident prone. And if that isn't enough, the fat toddler more often than not grows up into the fat school-ager who in turn becomes the obese adolescent. The fat toddler is not yet vulnerable to the painful emotional consequences of being overweight—but just wait until he's a fat school-ager!

THE TROUBLE WITH GIVING IN TO TODDLER'S DEMANDS

What else happens during toddlerhood that leads to faulty nutrition? For one thing, the child himself becomes more assertive and better able to indicate his likes and dislikes. "Every day in every way, Mark becomes more of a person," was the way one delighted mother put it. All parents are thrilled when their children begin to talk. It is an exciting time. As your toddler learns to use words, he naturally begins to *ask* for things. Most mothers and fathers have a strong desire to respond positively to these requests. That's great. But when parents respond positively to too many requests for cookies, soft drinks, and other so-called treats, as so many parents unfortunately do, that's not so great.

I am not as extreme in my views as some of my colleagues in this area of nutrition. I have seen no evidence to suggest that an occasional piece of candy, slice of cake, or dish of ice cream is harmful. These foods are not poison, and there is no reason at all for a healthy toddler not to have them occasionally. But I begin to worry about the toddler whose parents *always* give in to his demands for sweets, because I know what it leads to—

"treats" in excess kill the toddler's appetite for other more nutritious foods. At the same time an unhealthy snacking pattern is being established and the longer it continues the more difficult it will be to change it later on.

I continue to be amazed that in this enlightened age of nutrition there are still so many parents who are simply not aware that unlimited treats and junk foods are not good for a child. But believe me, such people, often very warm and loving parents, do exist. I can understand it when the unaware mother or father gives in consistently to a toddler's demands for high-calorie, high-sugar, high-salt, low-nutrition treats and snacks. But parents with a fairly sophisticated knowledge of nutrition also give their kids too much junk food. These parents probably think, "Why not give him what he wants? Why upset him? There's plenty of time in the future to worry about his health and his weight."

In one sense, they're absolutely right. There *will* be plenty of time in the future, but why wait for the problems to develop? You can protect your toddler simply by remembering these two points:

1. If you always give in now, when your child is a toddler, you will find it much more difficult to be firm in later years, when habits are even more difficult to correct.
2. You are not depriving your child of anything important when you place appropriate limits on treats and junk foods. Just the opposite. By taking a stand now you are acting in his best interest and there is no reason for you to feel guilty when you say no.

THE GREAT FOOD WARS

There is still another phenomenon that influences toddler nutrition. At about one year of age the child's rate of growth begins to slow. As his first-year growth spurt diminishes, so does his appetite. This is perfectly normal and predictable, but many parents, especially first-time parents, are completely unprepared for this. In fact, I have known quite a few who were thrown for a loop when they suddenly realized that their previously hungry infant, who used to enjoy just about every type of food offered, had suddenly turned into a finicky toddler who seemed to eat practically nothing.

This sets the stage for the start of the great food wars. Concerned because their little one refuses to eat as much as he did before, and convinced that he will become ill or even starve if he won't eat more, his parents will often spend long periods of time and great effort coaxing, cajoling, and even bribing him to clear his plate.

I wish I had a nickel (even in this age of inflation) for every time a parent has said, "If you don't eat your spinach, you can't have any cake." (Thus making spinach seem like a thoroughly detestable food while elevating cake to the highest desirability.) Your toddler probably still won't eat the spinach—he can be pretty stubborn—but he will get the cake anyway, as well as a few cookies at bedtime, because his parents need to reassure themselves that he's eaten *something*, and won't wake up starving during the night.

A scenario can develop in which a toddler who seemingly eats practically "nothing" actually takes in more calories than he needs over the course of a day. Those calories are likely to be "empty" ones, because they're supplied by treats and junk foods that are high in sugar (often also high in fat) but don't contain many of the essential nutrients needed for optimal growth.

EATING LESS IS NORMAL

The best advice I can give parents who worry when their toddler's appetite seems to disappear is to remind them that eating less is normal at this age. It is part of the body's way of adjusting to the toddler's slower growth rate. If he is healthy to begin with, it won't make him sick and he certainly won't waste away if he doesn't finish all the food on the plate. The toddler can get by with just a bite or two of this and a couple of bites of that at mealtimes, provided the food offered is nutritious, because he *really* does not need that large a quantity. A good piece of advice is to let your toddler's appetite decide how much or how little he eats and not what you think he should eat. This same advice holds true for children of all ages.

Your job as a parent is to make sure that the food he *does* get is good nutritious fare, and then let it go at that. No coaxing. No nagging. No bribing him to eat more than he wants. And no loading him up with sweets or junk food later on to make up for the meal he's missed. If he enjoys a snack between meals or before bedtime, as most toddlers do, offer something that supplies more than just "empty" sugar calories or calories loaded with too much salt or fat. You will find a list of healthful food snacks further along in this chapter.

Never force your toddler to eat. Not only will it probably not work, but it will turn food into an emotionally loaded issue and make mealtime tense and frustrating for the whole family. Let your child be the judge of how much food he eats at a sitting. Allow him to decide when he's had enough. If he gets hungry later on, take advantage—this is a golden opportunity and so use it to get something nutritious into his little tummy. Don't throw the opportunity away by offering him non-nutritious foods.

TOO LITTLE IRON

Studies have shown that one to three year olds are most prone to iron deficiency. The question is *why* in this land of plenty are so many toddlers iron deficient? This is an interesting question when one considers that iron is present in so many readily available foods. Part of the answer has to do with the changes that occur in a child's diet when he is switched from breast milk or formula and baby food to cow's milk and table food. This drastic change often occurs at one year of age. The small quantity of iron in breast milk is very well absorbed, and an iron-fortified formula meets the infant's needs for this mineral. As we pointed out in the previous chapter about the infant, iron intake is often augmented by baby cereal which, by law in the United States, must be fortified with iron. When breast milk or iron-fortified formula is stopped, the infant is immediately deprived of an important daily source of this mineral. Another good source of iron is removed from his diet when his parents replace baby cereal with an adult-type cereal, unless of course they choose an iron-fortified one.

At the same time the toddler's appetite begins to decrease. He often becomes a picky eater who turns down any number of good iron-rich foods. Already we can begin to see how iron deficiency might now develop. But there is more. Cow's milk, remember, contains practically no iron. But many toddlers, even the poor eaters, continue to enjoy their milk as much as ever, and milk is filling. When a toddler drinks lots of milk, there is no room or appetite left for other iron-containing foods.

With these facts in mind, I prescribe a daily iron-fortified vitamin for many of the toddlers in my practice.

There is another point to be made about iron deficiency. When it is combined with pica, the craving for nonfood substances (which is not uncommon among toddlers), the consequences can be very serious. Children with pica try to eat almost anything—dirt, old newspapers, paint, and plaster off the wall, all of which may contain quantities of lead. A child who is iron deficient absorbs lead more readily into his system. When enough lead is ingested and absorbed, lead poisoning develops, and with it irreparable brain damage may result. Preventing iron deficiency will help protect the toddler with pica from getting poisoned from lead.

USE YOUR INFLUENCE!

The switch to table food, the acquisition of language coupled with a growing assertiveness, and a decreased appetite are all part of a toddler's normal development. At the same time these factors easily can lead to nutritional imbalances and poor eating habits, the consequences of which can affect your child now and for the rest of his life. That is the bad news about toddlers.

Now here's the good news: Your power to shape your child's eating and exercise patterns is greater now than it ever will be in the future. Even though toddlers are notorious for their stubbornness (think of the terrible two's) and even though many of them display an ornery streak that makes it difficult to get them to do what you want them to do, where food and exercise are concerned, you the parents still have almost total control.

For these few years, outside influences remain minimal and your toddler will be almost completely dependent on you for what he eats. Now, when he spends most of every day with you or with a baby-sitter with whom you can leave specific feeding instructions, is the time to act. You may not be able to get him to eat all the vegetables you would like him to have, but don't nag or bribe him to eat. You *can* make sure that what he does eat is healthy and nutritious simply by not offering him the bad stuff.

Put small portions of vegetables on his plate without pressuring him to eat. In time, he may surprise you and actually eat some, especially if you offer a variety. Instead of cooking all the vegetables, see what happens if you offer some of them raw. I have seen many a toddler turn up their noses at cooked cabbage, for example, but who thought crisp raw cabbage was the greatest. It is amazing how often toddlers who were always nagged to eat their vegetables quickly learn to like them when the heat is off.

I give the same advice to parents whose children don't seem to like fruit or fish or anything else nutritious. Keep offering, but don't fight about it. It would be ideal if all toddlers would eat a large variety of foods, but the fact is that many of them won't.

Your child will not become malnourished if he does not eat everything you think he needs. Don't let your concern about what your child won't eat frighten you into giving him too much of the foods he *will* eat. The end result will certainly not be the weight stabilization you are aiming for.

Let me tell you about the mother of a markedly overweight eighteen month old who swore she wanted nothing more than to help her baby slim down. I gave her my usual pep talk, copies of appropriate toddler diets, and guidelines to proper exercise, and so on, and told her to bring her son back in a month. Well, a month later, when I weighed the child, he had gained 2½ pounds. "I thought you were going to follow the diet recommendations we discussed," I said to the mother. "I did," she protested, "but Tommy wouldn't eat the chicken, he wouldn't eat the fish, and he screamed when I put vegetables on his plate. I knew he wouldn't survive so I had to give him *something* to fill him up." The "something" she gave was cookies and two quarts of milk each day.

GOOD FOOD FOR EVERYONE

Other parents, when they follow the Eden menu plans for the fat toddler for the first time, look worried and say, "How can I expect my little child to eat this way, while the rest of the family has regular meals?" The answer to that one is you can't. It is unreasonable to expect a toddler—fat, thin, or in-between—to be happy with foods that do not look or taste like the stuff mom, dad, and brother Billy have on their plates. Nobody likes to feel discriminated against, including toddlers who have a natural desire to imitate their elders.

So, what is a parent to do? If you truly are serious about wanting to protect your child against the dangers of overweight and to give him all the present and future benefits of sound nutrition, you have two alternatives. In my view, only one of them makes sense. You could feed your toddler in a separate room or feed him at a different hour so he won't know his food is different from the rest of the family's. This approach makes no sense at all. I believe it is important for a family to eat together. Mealtime in this hectic day and age is often the *only* time that a family can be together and enjoy each others' company.

The other more sensible option is to modify the meals for the entire family so they're more like the Eden toddler diet. That means more fruits and vegetables, more fish and chicken, more whole-grains and less red meat, sugar, salt, fat, and cholesterol for *everyone*. This is one of life's future no-lose situations— better nutrition for all. Not only that, more than one mother has reported back to me that after switching her baby to the Eden diet program she and her husband (sometimes both) lost a few extra unneeded pounds without even trying. Who knows, maybe it will happen in your family too!

Our specific menu plans are designed for normal-weight toddlers. If your toddler is markedly overweight, refer to the daily menu plans on pages 216–220.

TODDLER DIET GUIDELINES

Don't worry too much if your toddler isn't 100 percent cooperative. He may not care to eat *everything* listed in the guidelines and menus. He may, for example, decide he doesn't like vegetables and refuse to eat some and even all varieties for a while. That's okay; don't force the issue. Continue to offer them and, if possible, vary the cooking methods from time to time, such as occasionally serving them raw. You will be pleasantly surprised when he discovers that some vegetables are not so awful and some of them even taste pretty good.

Remember that it is less important that he eats *all* the right things than that he doesn't eat *too much* of the wrong things.

If you are serious about wanting to change the way your toddler eats (and I hope that by now you are), you will probably have to make some changes in your own diet as well. Toddlers are notorious copycats and learn by example.

The guidelines: A varied diet offering foods from each of the basic four food groups is the best assurance of optimal nutrition.

I. Grains
1. Offer breads that are whole-grain or enriched such as whole wheat, rye, pumpernickel.
2. Use barley, buckwheat (kasha), corn meal, oatmeal, pasta, rice, and wheat.
3. Unsweetened dry breakfast cereals may be included but not to the exclusion of whole-grain or infant cereals.

II. Protein foods (including fish and legumes)

1. Encourage poultry, veal, fish (remove the bones), and legumes such as chick peas, lentils, and dry beans.
2. Limit red meats (pork, beef, lamb) trimmed of fat, to no more than three servings per week.
3. Peanut butter, a good protein food, may be offered occasionally instead of meat.
4. Restrict the number of eggs to 3–4 per week.
5. Avoid serving smoked, salted, cured, and delicatessen meats such as bacon, ham, bologna, corn beef, salami, frankfurters, and so on, except on very special occasions. These meats are high in fat and salt and many have high levels of nitrite preservatives. Nitrites have been found to cause cancer in laboratory animals, so it is best to eat as little of these compounds as possible.

III. Fruits/Vegetables

1. Offer a citrus fruit (orange, grapefruit, tangerine) or a glass of citrus juice daily.
2. Avoid juice or fruit drinks with added sugar.
3. Offer fruits often at snack time and as a dessert.
4. Include at least one serving per day of a bright yellow- or orange-colored vegetable (tomato, sweet potato, carrot, yellow squash, beets, etc.) and at least one of a leafy green vegetable (spinach, escarole, broccoli, cabbage, etc.)
5. Fresh vegetables are best and may be offered raw, or cooked but still crunchy.
6. Vegetables should not be fried in butter or other saturated fats.
7. Potatoes should be served boiled, mashed, or baked—not fried. Add low-fat milk and diet margarine or cottage cheese for added flavor.

IV. Milk and milk products

1. Limit milk to two to three glasses per day.
2. Use only low-fat or skim milk.
3. Offer yogurt and low-fat cheese as snacks.

HEALTHY SNACKS FOR TODDLERS

A mid-morning and mid-afternoon snack keep toddlers happy. These snacks are full of nutrition and low in refined sugars.

Fruit Juice (not drink), unsweetened:
  Orange
  Apple
  Grape
  Cranberry-apple

Vegetables and Fruits:
  Carrots grated or sticks
  Raisins (if yogurt covered, children think it's candy!)
  Apple slices
  Banana slices
  Orange sections
  Seedless grapes
  Date pieces
  Dried apples
  Dried apricots
  Melon slices

Grains:
  Whole-wheat crackers with farmer cheese or tuna salad
  Peanut butter on whole-wheat pita bread
  Cheese melted on whole-wheat pita bread
  Oatmeal cookies
  Unsalted pretzels
  Popcorn, unsalted, unbuttered
  Rice cakes with nut butter

Milk:
  Low-fat milk
  Low-fat yogurt
  Slice of cheese
  Frozen yogurt
  Ice-milk

MEAL PLANS FOR TODDLERS

The following is one week of specific meal plans for toddlers:

MONDAY

BREAKFAST	3 Tb. enriched farina cooked in water and ½ cup low-fat milk ½ cup orange juice
SNACK	2 graham crackers ½ cup low-fat milk
LUNCH	1 cup tomato soup made with ½ cup low-fat milk 1 small round (or ½ large round piece) whole-wheat pita bread 1 Tb. smooth peanut butter
SNACK	½ cup apple juice
DINNER	2 or 3 oz. dry fresh spinach noodles 4 Tbs. low-fat cheese sauce made with ¼ cup low-fat milk thickened with 1 Tb. flour, cooked, and added to 2 oz. American cheese ½ cup glazed carrots with 1 tsp. marmalade Cranberry-apple spritzer made with ½ cup cranberry juice ½ cup seltzer

TUESDAY

BREAKFAST	Scrambled eggs made with 2 egg whites, 1 egg yolk, and 1 oz. American cheese cooked in nonstick skillet

	1 slice whole-wheat bread 1 tsp. soft margarine ½ cup orange juice
SNACK	½ cup low-fat milk 1 small round whole-wheat pita bread 2 tsp. smooth peanut butter ½ tsp. jam
LUNCH	2 oz. dry noodles with ¼ cup cottage cheese 1 cup seedless grapes ½ cup low-fat milk
SNACK	½ banana
DINNER	2 stalks steamed broccoli 3 oz. skinless chicken breast, steamed ½ cup brown rice ½ cup apple juice 1 oatmeal cookie

WEDNESDAY

BREAKFAST	1 hard boiled egg ½ bagel with 1 oz. melted cheese ½ cup apple juice
SNACK	10 grapes
LUNCH	½ cup cottage cheese ½ cup sliced peaches 2 whole-wheat crackers ½ cup low-fat milk
SNACK	½ cup Indian pudding made with low-fat milk, molasses, and raisins
DINNER	1 cup split pea soup 2 wheat crackers 3 oz. sliced turkey

Tomato slices
1 Tb. Russian dressing
½ cup low-fat milk

THURSDAY

BREAKFAST	1 small bran muffin with 1 tsp. margarine ½ cup low-fat milk
SNACK	1 apple, sliced
LUNCH	1 slice whole-wheat bread with 1 Tb. peanut butter 1 tsp. preserves ½ cup low-fat milk
SNACK	½ cup sliced strawberries
DINNER	1 cup cooked spaghetti ½ cup cottage cheese 2 Tbs. petite peas ½ cup strawberry ice-milk

FRIDAY

BREAKFAST	½ ripe banana
	¼ cup low-fat vanilla yogurt
	1 slice whole-wheat toast with
	  1 tsp margarine
	2 graham crackers with
	  1 Tb. peanut butter and 2 tsp. jam
	½ cup apple juice

LUNCH	2 slices turkey breast 1 slice whole-wheat bread 1 Tb. mayonnaise ½ cup rice pudding ½ cup low-fat milk

SNACK	2 whole-wheat fig cookies ½ cup low-fat milk
DINNER	2 oz. broiled cod 3 Tbs. mashed sweet potatoes with ½ tsp. margarine 1 slice raisin bread with ½ tsp. margarine ½ orange, in sections ½ cup low-fat milk

SATURDAY

BREAKFAST	4 oz. orange juice 1 egg, scrambled 1 slice whole-wheat toast with 1 tsp. diet margarine ½ cup low-fat milk
SNACK	½ banana
LUNCH	1 cup chicken noodle soup 4 salt-free saltines with 1 oz. Swiss cheese 2 Tbs. sliced carrots ¼ cup Indian pudding ½ cup low-fat milk
SNACK	½ cup apple juice 2 molasses cookies
DINNER	3 oz. sliced chicken breast ½ cup egg noodles 2 Tbs. broccoli ½ cup low-fat yogurt 1 piece corn bread 1 tsp. margarine

SUNDAY

BREAKFAST	½ whole-wheat bagel 1 slice American cheese ½ cup unsweetened grape juice
SNACK	⅓ cup low-fat vanilla yogurt
LUNCH	3 oz. tunafish with 2 tsp. mayonnaise 1 slice whole-wheat bread Cucumber slices ½ cup tomato soup ½ cup low-fat milk
SNACK	10 grapes
DINNER	3 oz. lean hamburger 1 slice whole-wheat bread 2 tsp. catsup 2 Tb. green beans ½ cup orange juice ⅓ cup rice pudding made with low-fat milk

CHAPTER 11
Feeding Your Preschooler

Bigger and definitely better than ever! That's the way many parents of preschoolers view their children. Bigger, of course. The preschooler is still growing rapidly, although not nearly so fast as she did as a toddler. And better because the three-to-six-year-old child is typically less negative, less demanding, more cooperative and, in general, a much easier person to have around the house than when she was two or three. Unlike the toddler who was so busy learning how to assert her will and proclaim her individuality, the preschooler is more interested in conforming and doing things the "right" way. Developmentally, she is at the stage of striving to be more grown-up. In fact, few things are more disturbing to a four or five year old than to be called a baby. Because you, the parents, continue to be the most important grown-ups in her life, her role models, your child will be eager to do things your way, at least most of the time.

I certainly don't mean to imply that the typical preschooler is a little robot who can be programmed to do exactly as you tell her, or that she will model herself after you in every way. Some children are naturally less adaptable and more feisty at every stage along the way. Even the most cooperative and conforming preschooler will be balky and stubborn at times. But the overriding tendency at this age is for the child to watch and listen to her parents in order to emulate them.

This has important ramifications for your child's health and well-being. Children always need guidance, but they don't always want it. Preschoolers, at least most of them most of the time, do want and accept your guidance. Thus this is an ideal time to reinforce the good eating habits you encouraged in your child when she was a toddler. If, on the other hand, you have not up to now instilled correct eating patterns, this is the perfect time to start making changes for the better. Her childhood ways shape her future. The food habits your preschooler falls into now will influence her chances for a long and vigorously healthy life. Whether those influences are positive or negative is primarily up to you.

SAYING NO TO JUNK FOOD

In these early years your child is still almost totally dependent on you her parents for every single morsel of food. If her diet is a healthy one, it is because you made it so, by providing family meals that give her enough of the good things she needs and not too much of the bad things. Certainly, if you have been following the Eden diet plan nutritional guidelines (or similar guidelines), your child is off to an excellent start. The credit is all yours.

But if the family diet is typical of what most Americans eat— too high in calories, fat and cholesterol, refined sugar and salt, and too low in iron and fiber, your preschooler is already beginning to establish eating habits that could be hazardous to her future health. These habits contribute to the high rate of heart disease, high blood pressure, stroke, obesity, and some types of cancer found in our adult population. Parents must accept the responsibility for the potentially dangerous future consequences of such a diet.

If little four-year-old Robert sees his father pouring salt all over his food, then Robert, who at this age believes that daddy is better than Superman, and wants to be exactly like him, will learn to oversalt his food too. If mom does not like fish, and it is never served to the family, Robert will grow up viewing fish as a third-rate food. If big brother, Joseph, at age ten, eats bacon and two eggs for breakfast each morning, it won't be long before little Robert is doing the same. And so, right down the line with every kind of food that is served or not served in the house. The only outside influence that even begins to approach the power of parents in shaping preschooler food preferences is television. The TV influence on this age group is profound. When the toddler watches TV, she doesn't always understand what she sees and hears. The school-age child and adolescent usually can discriminate between entertainment and advertising messages, and in time actually develop a healthy criticism, but the preschooler is ripe for exploitation. She is old enough to understand the words and images but not sophisticated enough to realize she is being hustled. Candy, soft drinks, sugar-coated cereals, high-calorie, low-nutrition snacks, and fastfoods peddled on TV seem glamorous and irresistible to her. When the voice-over says, "Tell Mommy to run right out and get some today!" the preschooler can be counted on to do just that.

Now, giant food corporations and their advertising agencies are in the business of turning a profit. I don't agree with those who would like to ban these food commercials from the airways. After all, we are living in a free country and we still have freedom of choice. But there should be freedom of choice for parents as well as for advertisers. The food companies are free to try to sell their products to you and your children, but you are just as free to say *no* to the ads and to your preschooler's demands when it's appropriate.

Saying "no" to demands for food a child sees on TV or notices other people eating is an important skill many parents are unwilling or unable to develop in themselves, even in those clear-cut cases when "no" is the obvious answer. Saying "yes" is always easier because it avoids the parent-child conflict. If you have never learned the fine art of saying "no" to your preschooler's food demands, try to keep in mind that a firm stand is better for your child than giving in. If you establish firm ground rules, it will convince her that eating properly is important and that you care enough about her and what she eats to stick to your guns. Very few preschoolers understand a complicated discussion about nutrition and I won't encourage you to provide elaborate explanations of why you don't want her to eat such and such. But you can certainly make it clear that too much candy or too many potato chips, and so on, is not good for her and that you must for this reason say no. Try it. The first few times will be the most difficult. In time, if you remain consistent, your child will learn to accept these new ground rules. An occasional candy bar, for example, won't have a long-term negative impact on your preschooler's health. It is when these foods stop being treats and start becoming an everyday part of a child's diet that I worry.

Unfortunately, that is what has already happened with many of the preschoolers I see in my office. They come in munching cookies or candy of various kinds. I rarely see them eating an apple, carrot sticks, or yogurt, all of which would be much healthier and just as easy for a parent to bag. When I question mothers and fathers about their preschooler's diet or when I ask them to bring me a food diary listing everything their children eat for several days, my suspicions are confirmed. Sweetened drinks and low-nutrition, high-calorie, high-salt and sugar snacks are *not* saved for special occasions in many families. Rather, these foods are already an integral part of the everyday diet of their preschoolers.

Here is what four-year-old Amanda ate on a typical day, according to the food diary faithfully kept by her mother:

7:00 A.M.
Orange juice
Presweetened cereal and milk

9:00 A.M.
2 chocolate chip cookies
Milk

12:00 noon
Cream cheese and jelly sandwich on white bread
Chocolate cookie
Milk

2:00 P.M.
Cupcake
Sweetened fruit drink

3:30 P.M.
Ice pop (strawberry)

5:00 P.M.
Salted corn chips (½ bag)

6:30 P.M.
Hot dog on roll
Mashed potatoes
Applesauce
Milk

8:00 P.M.
2 chocolate chip cookies
Sweetened fruit drink

Let's see what Amanda ate that day:

Two servings of fruit (orange juice and applesauce)
One serving of vegetable (the mashed potato)
Three servings of milk
One serving of meat (the hot dog)

So far, not *too* bad, although it could be better. However, with the addition of the presweetened cereals, the chocolate chip and chocolate cookies, the cream cheese, the sweetened fruit drinks, the ice pop, and the corn chips, this child's diet turns out to be much too high in calories, fat, and sugar, and too low in essential nutrients. The ratio of "treats" to healthy, nutritious foods is way out of proportion.

As a parent, you can make all the difference by feeding your preschooler the type of diet that will enhance her chances for better health now or for the rest of her life, or, put another way, at this stage of your child's life, you are the *only* one who can make a difference. After all, your preschooler is still too young to select, buy, and cook her own food. She has no control over what appears on her plate, but *you do*.

Later on, of course, the situation will change. She will be spending more and more time away from home at school and visiting friends. She will have an allowance and with money in her pocket will be more independent. With this money she will be capable of going to the local candy store for all sorts of "treats" and, as she continues to mature, she will become less receptive to your ideas about what is and what isn't healthy. In fact, years from now when your child reaches adolescence you may discover that the best way to get her to do *anything* is to tell her to do just the opposite. The time to make nutritional changes is *now*.

Every once in a while when I encourage the mother of one of my young patients to modify her child's diet for the better, the response will be, "But Jenny doesn't like vegetables," or, "Whenever I serve fish, she just leaves it on her plate." To which my answer always is, it's less important to get your child to eat large amounts of the good stuff than it is to prevent her from becoming habituated to the bad stuff. It would be great if Jenny loved vegetables and broiled fish, but don't worry if she turns them down. Preschoolers do not have large appetites and, in fact, need much less food than most parents imagine. Needing very little food to feel satisfied, it is natural that a child this age often picks and chooses from the different items on her plate. Don't worry about it. If she has one or two servings of fruit each day, it won't matter much if she ignores her vegetables. If she eats a slice of cheese or some yogurt at snack time or lunch, it won't be a tragedy if she refuses fish or chicken at dinner.

The key to feeding your child well now and helping her to develop proper food habits for a lifetime is to stop worrying about what she doesn't eat and instead make sure that the food she *does* eat is nutritious.

It is important not to force any child to eat when she doesn't feel like it. Further, don't tell your child that it makes you sad and unhappy when she doesn't finish her vegetables. Don't make her feel guilty by pointing out how hard you worked preparing the meal. Don't make comments equating food and love such as: "If you really love mommy, you will finish everything on your plate." Above all, never bribe her with promises of a special dessert or an after-dinner treat if she'll finish her milk. All of these ploys make food an emotional issue loaded with psychological overtones it should not have.

If your preschooler sees you enjoying vegetables, fish, chicken, lean meat, fruits, and whole-grain products, chances are she too will soon learn to enjoy them. It won't matter if she does not eat *everything*. By providing a wide variety of good foods from which she can choose and try, and limiting the foods that can eventually cause problems, you will be helping your preschooler get a head start toward optimal health and fitness.

WATCH CHOLESTEROL AND FAT

In advising parents to limit their preschoolers' intake of highly saturated, high-cholesterol foods, I sometimes use the traffic safety analogy. It goes something like this: Even though it will be a few more years before your child is old enough to cross streets by herself, you probably have already begun to talk to her about traffic lights and looking both ways for cars before stepping off the curb. You do this to impress on her the need for caution and to lay the groundwork for future good safety habits. There is no way for you to know for sure whether these efforts will keep her from being hurt by a passing car when she gets older, but you teach her anyway. You realize that if you don't, her chances of being run over will be greater.

In the same way, limiting the saturated fat and cholesterol content of your child's diet now is a safety measure. Preschoolers are not at risk for heart attack or stroke or the nutrition-related cancers that are linked to a highly saturated, high-cholesterol diet. Nevertheless, it is extremely important to establish "safe" eating habits in the early years in order to avoid problems later on. There is no guarantee that the correct diet started now and continued throughout adulthood will prevent those just-mentioned killer diseases, but we *do* know that the wrong diet increases the chances of becoming a victim.

One young couple seemed relieved and even pleased when I suggested that they switch their preschooler, Jennifer, age four, to a diet lower in saturated fat and cholesterol. Most parents groan and complain when I urge them to modify their child's diet; they realize that these changes won't be easy. This wife hastened to explain: "My husband must restrict his cholesterol and fat intake. Since we thought his diet might be harmful for Jennifer, I began cooking double meals—low cholesterol and fat for us and "ordinary" food for Jennifer. Now that you have told us that the lower cholesterol and lower-fat eating will also help Jennifer, I can go back to cooking the same food for all of us!"

IRON FOR BETTER BEHAVIOR

Not long ago a perplexed mother described her five year old's behavior as follows: "She is irritable and at nursery school she can't seem to concentrate on learning. At home she mopes and sits around. Donna just doesn't have the get-up-and-go of her older brother, Louis." I carefully examined Donna, but found nothing physically wrong. Then I questioned her mother about the foods she ate. "No, she rarely eats fruits or vegetables," she said. "We're meat and potatoes and she also eats spaghetti. Oh, she really *loves* her milk."

"Let's see what happens if you cut down on her milk, offer her more leafy green vegetables and an iron-fortified cereal, and put her on a multivitamin with iron," I said. She looked doubtful but assured me she would give it a try. I did not see or hear from her for several weeks, when she brought Donna in so I could have a look at her toe, which she thought might have broken when she fell off her tricycle. I examined her toe (it wasn't broken) and then asked how Donna was behaving lately. "You know, Doctor, Donna does seem more energetic and alert these days," she answered. "I don't know what's in those vegetables or in the vitamins, but she is a different girl now."

To be perfectly honest, I am not sure that eating the leafy green vegetables and taking the iron supplement actually were what altered Donna's behavior for the better. I didn't test her for iron deficiency, but I do know this: Insufficient amounts of iron in a child's diet can produce the symptoms described by this mother on her previous visit to my office. From what she told me about her daughter's diet I suspected that she was not getting enough iron. Was the iron responsible for the change? There is no way to prove that it was (although I could have tried by ordering some blood tests before and after), yet the evidence seemed to point in that direction.

PRESCHOOL DIET GUIDELINES

The Eden diet guidelines and meal plans for preschool-age children is consistent with the low-fat, low-cholesterol guidelines recently issued by both the American Heart Association and the American Cancer Society. By having her follow the Eden diet plan now you will be reducing her adult risk for heart attack, stroke, high blood pressure, and some nutrition-related cancers. You will also be shielding her from the dangers associated with obesity and iron deficiency.

Your preschooler does not need to eat all of the recommended foods in the suggested amounts to reap the benefits of better eating. She may decide she does not want vegetables one day or refuse her chicken or fish on another day. This is no cause for alarm. Don't force the issue. Do continue to offer a wide variety of foods and, if possible, vary the cooking methods and seasonings from time to time. Keep in mind that children this age tend to like their food plain and simple. (For example, it's not unusual for a preschooler to turn up her nose at a mixed salad, but to enjoy a wedge of lettuce and a slice of tomato if they are served separately.)

Remember, at this age your child is concerned with becoming more grown-up and because you are the primary adult role model in her life, your influence can have a positive effect on the way she eats. If your own eating habits leave something to be desired, now is the time for you to make changes for the better. The Eden diet will benefit you as much as it will your preschooler.

The following are some important Eden diet guidelines for you to observe in planning your preschooler's meals:

1. Use low-fat or skim milk and keep the total daily intake to a maximum of three glasses.
2. Offer whole-grain breads whenever possible.
3. Use dry unsweetened breakfast cereals, preferably iron fortified. Don't add sugar to cereal, but use fresh fruit instead.
4. Encourage poultry, veal, and fish and limit red meats, trimmed of fat, to no more than three servings per week.
5. Use no more than three to four egg yolks per week.
6. Cut out or at least cut down on smoked, salted, cured, or deli meats.
7. Offer fresh fruit as dessert and as between-meal snacks.
8. Use fresh vegetables whenever possible (may be offered raw).
9. Use natural unsweetened fruit juices and keep sweetened soda out of the house.
10. Keep the salt shaker off the table.

HEALTHY SNACKS FOR PRESCHOOLERS

Always keep a few of these healthy snacks on hand for your preschooler. (Also see Snacks for Toddlers.)

Fruits and vegetables
Orange slices
Apple wedges
Seedless grapes
Carrot sticks
Zucchini sticks
Pineapple chunks
Banana chunks
Cherry tomatoes stuffed with cottage cheese
Applesauce with Grape-Nuts or wheat germ

Beverages
Banana cooler (made with low-fat milk blended with honey and a half banana)
Fruit juice, unsweetened
Sherbet floats made with fruit juice
Peanut cow (skim milk blended with peanut butter)
Vanilla ice milk—grape juice float
Fruit juice spritzer (seltzer with fruit juice)

Grains
Whole-grain crackers with:
  Natural peanut butter
  Cottage cheese
  Low-fat cheese
Bran muffins
Homemade pizza on whole-wheat English muffins
Whole-wheat pita round with peanut butter

Frozen goodies
Frozen banana rolled in chopped nuts
Frozen yogurt on a stick
Frozen grapes or blueberries
Ice-milk with berries
Sherbet with crushed pineapple

½ cup raisin bran

MEAL PLANS FOR PRESCHOOLERS

The following are seven days of specific meal plans for normal weight preschoolers, including portion sizes:

MONDAY

BREAKFAST
½ cup Raisin Bran
1 cup low-fat (1%) milk
½ banana

SNACK	4 graham crackers ½ cup low-fat (1%) milk

LUNCH	Cheese sandwich
	   2 slices Muenster cheese
	   1 tsp. mayonnaise
	   1 tsp. mustard
	   2 slices whole-wheat bread
	   Lettuce and tomato
	½ cup apple juice
	Carrot sticks (1 carrot)
	Baked apple with 2 tsp maple syrup

DINNER	Oven-baked chicken (2 thighs, skinless) 1 ear corn on the cob ¾ cup brown rice 1 tsp. margarine ½ cup orange juice
SNACK	½ cup low-fat vanilla yogurt ½ cup strawberries

TUESDAY

BREAKFAST	1 corn muffin 1 tsp. margarine (soft) ½ pear, sliced 1 cup low-fat (1%) milk
LUNCH	Chicken salad—3 oz. chicken breast slices mixed with 1 Tb. mayonnaise ½ cup grapes—seedless grapes cut in half 2 slices rye bread 1 cup apple juice

SNACK	Banana Smoothee made with
	   ½ banana
	   ½ cup low-fat (1%) milk
	   2 tsp. honey
	   2 ice cubes

DINNER	Chinese beef with vegetables made with: 3 oz. lean flank steak, thinly sliced and sauteed with garlic and wedges of broccoli, carrots, onions, and red pepper strips in 2 tsp. olive oil ¾ cup brown rice ½ cup orange juice
SNACK	¾ cup strawberry ice-milk ¼ cup blueberries

WEDNESDAY

BREAKFAST	1 small bran muffin 1 Tb. peanut butter 1 cup low-fat milk
SNACK	1 cup low-fat blueberry yogurt

LUNCH	1 cup split pea soup
	English muffin pizza made with
	    1 English muffin
	    ¼ cup tomato sauce
	    2 oz. part-skim mozzarella cheese
	½ cup apple juice

DINNER	Stir-fried chicken and vegetables
	    3 oz. chicken
	    1 cup broccoli
	    1 Tb. safflower oil
	    2 tsp. teriyaki sauce
	    Garlic and ginger
	    ½ cup brown rice
	    ½ cup pineapple chunks
	1 uncoated frozen yogurt pop

SNACK	½ cup vanilla pudding made with low-fat milk

THURSDAY

BREAKFAST	1 small blueberry muffin with 1 tsp margarine ½ cup pineapple chunks ½ cup low-fat milk
LUNCH	1 cup egg noodles mixed with ½ cup cottage cheese 1 baked apple made with 1 tsp. honey and dash of cinnamon ½ cup orange juice
SNACK	1 cup low-fat fruit yogurt

DINNER	3 oz. lean ground beef cheeseburger:
	  ½ whole-wheat roll
	  1 Tb. catsup
	  1 oz. cheddar cheese
	½ cup baked beans
	1 medium baked potato with 2 Tbs. sour cream
	½ cup low-fat milk

SNACK	½ cup stewed prunes with 3 Tbs. low-fat milk

FRIDAY

BREAKFAST	¾ cup oatmeal made with
	  1 cup low-fat milk
	  2 Tbs. raisins
	1 cup apple juice

LUNCH	Macaroni and cheese made with
	  2 cups cooked macaroni
	  2 oz. shredded cheddar cheese
	3 Tbs. green beans
	10 frozen grapes
	1 cup low-fat milk

SNACK	1 rice cake with 2 tsp. peanut butter

DINNER	3 oz. pan-fried flounder made with
	    3 Tbs. bread crumbs
	    1 egg white
	    "fried" in 1 Tb. olive oil
	⅓ cup broccoli
	½ cup brown rice
	tomato slices with 1 Tb. Russian dressing
	Low-fat milk
	1 slice raisin bread with 1 tsp. margarine

SNACK	½ cup ice-milk with sliced strawberries

SATURDAY

BREAKFAST	¾ cup farina, cooked with
	    ½ cup low-fat milk
	    2 Tbs. chopped dates
	1 orange
	1 slice cracked-wheat toast with
	    1 tsp. margarine

LUNCH	Turkey and cheese sandwich
	    1 slice rye bread with
	    2 oz. turkey breast
	    1 oz. Swiss cheese
	    1 Tb. Russian dressing
	    tomato slices
	¼ cup carrot salad made with
	    1 Tb. mayonnaise
	    2 Tbs. raisins
	Grape soda made with
	    ½ cup grape juice
	    ½ cup seltzer

SNACK	1 small banana muffin with 2 tsp. peanut butter 1 cup low-fat milk

DINNER	1 cup noodles with
	   2 oz. tunafish, drained
	   3 Tbs. cottage cheese
	   3 Tbs. peas
	1 orange, sliced
	¾ cup cranberry juice

SNACK	½ frozen banana rolled in
	   1 Tb. orange juice
	   1 Tb. wheat germ

SUNDAY

BREAKFAST	1 whole-grain waffle ¼ cup low-fat vanilla yogurt ½ cup blueberries 1 Tb. syrup ½ cup orange juice
LUNCH	1 cup chunky vegetable soup 2 rice cakes with 4 Tbs. cottage cheese ½ cup unsweetened grape juice 1 small wedge cantaloupe

DINNER	3 oz. pork chops, pan-fried in 1 tsp. margarine
	¼ cup green beans
	½ cup mashed potatoes made with
	   1 tsp. margarine
	   2 Tbs. low-fat milk
	½ cup unsweetened applesauce
	½ cup low-fat milk

SNACK	1 small carrot-raisin muffin, spread with 1 tsp. honey ½ cup low-fat milk
SNACK	1 oz. peanuts

CHAPTER 12
Feeding Your Active School-Ager

In a sense we can say that the child of six has entered the "age of reason." His main job for the next few years will be to go to school and learn more and more about the world and about how it works. In addition to school itself, the six to ten year old will often be involved in school-sponsored extracurricular clubs, activities, and athletics, and may take classes of one kind or another, such as music or ballet after school hours.

As if this whirlwind of activity were not enough, the schoolager also wants to spend as much time as possible with friends. With school, homework, extracurricular activities, and friends, it all adds up to fewer hours spent at home.

During these years your child will be taking the first real steps toward independence. You as parents are still the primary people in his life, but whereas at age four or five he wanted nothing so much as to be just like you, now others are gaining in influence. Peer pressures get stronger and his teachers become more important with every passing year. This is natural and as it should be. But as his horizons continue to expand and as he spends more and more time away from the home, you will have less control over the important matters of diet and exercise.

If you encouraged healthy eating and exercise during the earlier stages of his life, those positive patterns are probably firmly established as habit by now. In effect, you have "immunized" him against the exaggerated food cravings and the sedentary lifestyle that contribute to the high rates of obesity, heart disease, stroke, and nutrition-related cancers afflicting our population. If this be the case, my congratulations to you! But this does not mean that you can simply sit back and relax. As your child continues to grow, he will be exposed to more and more outside influences, not all of them positive. You will need to keep up the good work at home to help offset some of these negative influences.

Based on my experience as a pediatrician, parents who made sure that their kids ate properly and had plenty of exercise opportunities as toddlers and preschoolers usually don't have problems keeping their children on track when they enter school. The key to it all is an on-going commitment and a home environment that continues to emphasize a healthy diet and plenty of exercise.

It is more difficult to change and modify bad habits than it is to reinforce good ones. But it *can* be done and it is never too late to begin. The evidence is all around us: men and women in their forties, fifties, and even sixties, cutting back on fat and cholesterol, eating less sugar and salt, getting more fiber into their diets, and embarking on brave new exercise programs—all with the specific aim of increasing their chances of living longer and healthier lives. If this group of adults can change habits that have evolved and become ingrained over decades, then so can your school-age child adapt to new styles of eating and exercise. If they have been raised up to this point in their lives on unhealthy diets and inadequate exercise, change is not only possible but it is a *must*, if you want your school-ager to have the benefits of better health now and for the rest of his life.

SCHOOL-AGE NUTRITION: WHAT IS IT ALL ABOUT?

What does your school-age child eat over the course of an average day? I have asked that question time and time again of parents, and time and time again the answer is: "You know, Dr. Eden, I'm really not sure."

Of course, parents usually know what their children eat at the evening meal when the whole family is gathered at the table. But that is only one meal out of three. Why is there such uncertainty about the other meals? If one considers the daily routine of most households, the answer becomes clear.

To begin with, many school-agers forage for their own breakfasts and eat them alone and on the run. Even when a parent is on hand in the morning, this important meal is usually choked down amidst the confusion that takes place when various family members are rushing to get to school or work on time. Under these circumstances, a parent may not pay enough attention to what goes into his or her child's stomach at the start of the day.

As for lunch, very few schools send children home for this meal nowadays, because it is no longer assumed that there is a mother waiting at home with a hot meal on the stove. Instead, almost all school-agers either bring a bag lunch or eat the lunch served in the school cafeteria. But either way it is difficult for parents to know what their children actually eat. The child who brings his lunch, for example, might indeed eat all of it or only some, or on occasion trade it away entirely for somebody else's lunch. I remember discussing this with a mother of an overweight nine year old. I raised the question of whether or not Robert was exchanging his nutritious, low-calorie lunch for a different, less healthy meal. On the next visit I was told that my suspicions were fairly accurate. It turned out that Robert did not exchange lunches with a friend but rather traded them away each day in exchange for two candy bars. If a child buys the school lunch, he may choose only those items he wants, even if he is forced to take everything on the school menu, and he can still eat selectively—for example, milk and dessert only.

After-school snacks may or may not be a mystery, depending on whether there is a parent or sitter at home in the afternoon. The latch-key child has the run of the kitchen and unless his parents have been very specific about what he may or may not have at this time, he will search the refrigerator and cupboards until he finds something to his liking.

And so it is not at all surprising that many parents are in the dark about what their school-agers eat on a typical day—and that many school-agers eat so poorly. If the scenario just described sounds familiar and if you want to give your child all the benefits of improved nutrition, you must first gain a greater degree of control over what he eats. This is difficult but not impossible. Let us go back over the day meal-by-meal and see what you can do to improve the situation.

BREAKFAST, LUNCH, DINNER, AND BEYOND

The best way to insure that your school-ager eats a good breakfast is for you to cook and serve a well-balanced, nutritious meal and insist that the whole family sit down together. The idea is to make breakfast as relaxed and enjoyable as possible. This may mean that everyone must get up 15 minutes earlier but believe me, it will be well worth it. With a good breakfast under his belt your child will feel and work better in school all morning long. Just as important, he will be less inclined to stop off on the way to school for a junk food snack. In my neighborhood I see kids stopping off at a candy store near school before the first bell rings. Some favorite purchases to start their day are potato chips or those little plastic-wrapped cakes washed down with a Coke or Pepsi, and this before nine o'clock in the morning!

A good breakfast does not have to be elaborate. It can be as simple as citrus fruit or juice, cereal (not the sugar-coated kind) with low-fat milk, a piece of whole-grain toast topped off with a cup of low-fat milk. Your job is to make healthy food available in a pleasant and relaxed setting. Even if he eats only a few bites they will be nutritious bites. When the goal is to upgrade your child's diet, follow this rule: Don't worry about the food he does not eat, just make sure that the food he does eat at home is healthy and nutritious.

It would be ideal if your child could come home from school for lunch. He would benefit from the exercise and you would be able to offer him a complete well-balanced meal. But because lunch at home is usually not possible, the next-best way is to pack a lunch. A sandwich is fine. The filling can be chicken, fish, lean red meat, peanut butter, or an egg (remember to limit total egg consumption to three to four per week). Use wholegrain bread. Include low-fat milk or juice, raw vegetables such as carrots or celery sticks, and a piece of fruit for dessert. That's it. No surprise treats such as candy, potato chips, cookies, or cake. No soft drinks. Your child may not eat everything you pack for him, and that is okay. Whatever portion of his lunch he *does* eat will be a nutritional *plus*, not a minus.

What about the child trading his excellent nutritious lunch for candy or cookies or cake? What can be done about it? I am afraid that I have no magic answer, no infallible strategy for putting an end to the practice of food swapping. I am sure of this, however: Your child will do less trading if you pack the foods that he truly likes. The previous sandwich guidelines allow you a wide range of choices, and I am sure that at least some of them will be acceptable.

Edward is eight years old with very finicky food tastes—about the only food that he liked was tunafish. He was a food swapper except when his mother made him a tunafish sandwich. The solution in that case was easy. I told Edward's mother that there was no reason that he could not have tunafish for every school-day lunch, five times a week. Of course you should always make it clear that you expect your child to eat the food you pack and not trade it with others. If you prepare and pack favorite foods and let him know how you feel about trading, he will stick with his lunch—at least most of the time.

After-school snacks present other difficulties, but these too can be minimized. Whoever is at home when your child returns from school should offer only healthy snacks, such as fruit, low-fat milk, and the items that you can find on the nutritious snack list later on in this chapter.

If he usually comes home to an empty house, simply stock up on these healthy snacks and keep them in a place that is easy for him to reach. It is also a good idea to leave a note on the refrigerator door suggesting an appropriate snack and where to find it. Just as important is not to have the unhealthy popular snack foods anywhere in the house. Self-control and will power are not the strongest points in the school-ager's makeup.

What if your child has become used to junk food snacks and will not eat the healthy foods when they are offered? I think that by now you can guess my answer. It makes no sense to try to pressure him. In fact, the less you react, the better. If your school-ager is hungry enough, he will eat. If he refuses the nutritious foods you have made available and holds out instead for junk foods, it's because he really isn't terribly hungry. Most important, don't give in and offer the junk food when your child turns up his nose at the good stuff. Naturally, it will be much easier to resist his demands for high-calorie, low-nutrition snacks if they're not in the house.

Most school-age children go off to school with an allowance. To those parents who are concerned about upgrading their children's nutrition, the money in the pocket presents problems because it allows the child to buy what I consider undesirable snack foods. Many parents feel uncomfortable about placing restrictions on what a child can buy with money that is his to do with as he pleases. I can understand these feelings although I don't agree with them. I believe that good nutrition is more important at this stage of a child's life than his absolute freedom to spend. Certainly if your school-ager is overweight, you must limit the amount of money he can spend on those foods that will only add to his weight problems.

If you are serious about wanting your school-ager to eat better, it makes good sense to go on record and tell him that you don't want him to spend his allowance on junk food. You can even go a step further and sit down together to work out a reasonable budget. See whether the two of you can arrive at a realistic estimate of how much money he needs for school supplies, how much for movies, how much for savings, and then tailor his allowance so that it is just a little more than he needs to cover his expenses. Maybe he will spend the extra money on junk food and maybe he won't. But at least there won't be enough left over to make a significant negative impact on his diet. It's certainly worth a try.

Dinner, the main meal of the day, is the one over which you

have the most control. Make it really count by serving an Eden diet—low in cholesterol and saturated fat, low in sugar and salt, high in iron, fiber, vitamins, and other essential nutrients. Need I add that such a diet offers the same benefits to younger and older brothers and sisters as well as to you, the parents? Don't force your child to eat anything he does not want, no matter how nutritious it is for him. The dinner table is no place for fighting, arguing, and ill will.

If you have bribed your child with food in the past, for example, promising a chocolate bar as a reward for eating his spinach, or threatened to withhold dessert as punishment for misbehavior, you should put a stop to these practices right now. It is important that your child view food simply as a means of satisfying hunger and not as a tool by which people can manipulate each other.

SCHOOL-AGERS, FAT, AND CHOLESTEROL

"Dr. Eden, how can I tell if Jay is getting too much fat and cholesterol in his diet?" asked a worried mother of one of my ten-year-old patients. I am asked this question a lot and I usually answer it with a series of questions of my own.

Does he drink whole milk and plenty of it?
Does he eat more than three or four eggs a week?
Do you slather butter (not margarine) on his vegetables and bread?
At family meals, do you almost always include fatty red meats such as beef, lamb, pork, or ham?
Do you give him large quantities of fried foods and greasy snack foods and treats?
Or, in other words, have you been feeding him the typical American diet?

If the answer to most or all of these questions is yes, there is no doubt in my mind that your school-ager is eating more fat and cholesterol than is good for him.

Medical researchers have concluded that for children aged five through eighteen, a blood cholesterol level of 110 mg/dL is "ideal." But in a study conducted by the American Health Foundation with support from the National Institutes of Health, it was found that the mean total blood cholesterol levels of a group of 1,500 fourth graders from Westchester County, New York was 166 mg/dL, and for a large group of fourth graders from the Bronx, New York, it was 173 mg/dL. In other words, the Westchester children had developed cholesterol levels that were on average 56 points higher and the Bronx youngsters' cholesterol levels 63 points higher than considered "ideal" for their age group.

The children from Westchester were predominantly white, from middle- and upper-income homes. Of the 2,000 Bronx youngsters studied, over 50 percent were minority youngsters, 45 percent white, and all were from low-income homes. Although these two groups live in the same part of the country, they represent a pretty good cross section of American children, and at an average age of nine, their blood cholesterol levels were already much too high!

Now that you know which foods are harmful in excess and why, you can do something about it. That "something" of course is to reduce the amount of fat and cholesterol your child eats each day by offering him less of the foods that are high in animal fat. The changes in the diet that reduce cholesterol levels in the blood are simple and easy to implement: Substitute low-fat or skim milk for whole milk, use margarine instead of butter, replace fatty red meats with fish or chicken as often as possible, limit eggs to three to four per week, and cut back on fried foods and greasy snacks. That really is all you have to do to help your school-ager grow up free of one of the major risk factors in cardiovascular disease. Needless to say, if the whole family switches to this low-fat, low-cholesterol eating, everyone will come out ahead.

"You mean to tell me if my six-year-old little boy eats less fat and cholesterol from now on he will never have a heart attack?" asked a skeptical young father. His question raises an important point. Diet isn't the only factor in determining who will have a heart attack or stroke and who won't. Among the other risk factors are family history, obesity, diabetes, cigarette smoking, and lack of exercise. Each of these conditions increases the likelihood of becoming a heart attack or stroke victim. When two or more of these factors are present, the risks increase dramatically. But in limiting your child's intake of fat and cholesterol, you are indirectly helping to remove not just one but two other risk factors—obesity and diabetes. In addition to getting his cholesterol down, you are also helping to protect him against obesity, because diet tends to be lower in calories. If his weight remains normal, he is less likely to develop diabetes as an adult.

There are few sure things in life and no one should be foolish enough to state categorically that dietary changes will completely protect your child from all kinds of illnesses. On the other hand, there is virtually no disagreement among researchers, practicing physicians, and public health officials, that keeping cholesterol levels low during childhood can go a long way in preventing problems later on.

This same low-fat, low-cholesterol diet can also reduce the chances of developing cancer of the breast and colon. These two dreaded and common types of cancer (as well as the equally virulent cancer of the prostate) appear to be linked to excess fat and cholesterol in the diet, and so the American Cancer Society has recently come out strongly in favor of low fat, low-cholesterol eating. In addition, the Cancer Society recommends increased consumption of vegetables, fruits, and high-fiber foods such as whole grains as further protection against some types of cancer. The more we learn about nutrition, the clearer it becomes that there is a *single* best way to eat—and reducing fat and cholesterol is a very important part of it.

IS YOUR SCHOOL-AGER IRON–RICH?

So far I have characterized the nutritional problems that can interfere with your child's optimal health and development as problems of *excess*, getting too much of the bad things. In the

United States today there is one important common nutritional *deficiency*, one element that large numbers of school-agers (and adults as well) need more of—namely, *iron* (see Chapter 5).

However, as a pediatrician, when I see a child who shows a marked lack of interest in his surroundings, is uncooperative or disruptive, who seems unusually tired, whose attention span is brief, or whose intellectual performance is not up to par, one of the areas I begin to consider as a possible cause of his symptoms is iron deficiency.

Iron is not hard to come by. It is not "rare" in the sense that it is supplied by only a limited number of exotic foods. The school-ager does not need enormous amounts of iron to remain iron sufficient. Boys (and girls until they begin to menstruate) require only about 8 milligrams per day. In fact, any child who eats a fairly well balanced diet should be iron sufficient, yet a large percentage of youngsters between the ages of six and ten get less than they need of this important nutrient. How do we explain this state of affairs?

In part, the answer is that many of the foods that are excellent sources of iron are not especially well liked by school-agers, while many of their favorite foods supply little or no iron. Your child probably enjoys red meat, which is a good source of iron, but how often does he cry out for other iron-rich foods such as prune juice, escarole, or liver? Now, what about his reaction to iron-poor foods such as pizza, French fries, ice cream, and cake? Need I say more?

Children with poor appetites are particularly at risk to become iron deficient because they don't eat much of anything. Children of school age with poor appetites who drink milk or juice with their meals are at even greater risk. With these kids there is a tendency to fill up on the beverage which then kills any appetite they might have had for the meal proper.

If your child is a poor eater who is accustomed to drinking milk or juice with his meals, one of the most important steps you can take to insure that he gets more iron is to stop offering any drink other than plain water at mealtimes. It is a simple strategy, so simple that many parents doubt it can be effective until they try it. Believe me, I have had many good reports from parents whose school-agers' appetites perked up considerably when the practice of serving milk or juice with the meal was stopped.

Some parents worry that their children won't get enough milk at mealtimes. As one mother put it, "Fred only drinks a couple of glasses of milk between meals and certainly that is not enough at his age." This mother, like many many others, has an unrealistic idea about how much calcium her child really needs. In truth, three glasses of milk per day supplies more than enough for the growing school-ager. Two glasses of milk plus some cheese or yogurt, or a serving of broccoli or spinach, does it as far as calcium is concerned. Let me mention now that there is no difference in the calcium content of whole milk, low-fat milk, or skim milk. The Eden diet uses only low-fat and skim milk because whole milk is too high in fat.

Even if your child's appetite leaves nothing to be desired, he still won't get the iron he needs each day if you don't serve enough of the iron-rich foods. Keep in mind also that many breakfast cereals are fortified with iron. Since most school-agers eat cereal, it is an excellent idea to routinely serve an iron-fortified brand. Read the nutritional information on the cereal box to make sure that the cereal you are buying really contains the added iron.

Once an iron-deficient child begins to get enough of this essential element, the symptoms associated with the deficiency often show marked improvement within a relatively short period of time. However, I don't want to raise unrealistic expectations. If your school-ager is iron deficient, correcting the condition won't turn him into a high-dynamo with the disposition of an angel and the high IQ of an Einstein, but you might well notice that he is less fatigued, less cranky, or can deal better with schoolwork.

In 1982 Dr. E. Pollitt and his colleagues gave a brief learning task to two groups of children—one group iron sufficient and one group iron deficient. The results showed that the iron-deficient group did measurably less well. This iron-deficient group of children was given an iron supplement for twelve weeks and then the two groups were retested. This time both groups performed equally well, proving once again that iron deficiency can interfere with learning.

Of course, not all school-agers in the United States are iron deficient. If you have been serving a wide variety of foods all along and your child is a good eater, the chances are excellent that he has been getting enough of this essential nutrient. In such a case, giving additional iron will not have any effect on his behavior or performance. On the other hand, if you have served the same foods over and over again and these foods fall into the iron-poor category, or if your youngster is a finicky eater, there is a real possibility that he is not getting the amount of iron he needs to remain truly fit and able to function at his best. In such a situation, additional iron could make a big difference.

The Eden diet includes a range of iron-rich foods that the six to ten year old will enjoy. If, however, your school-ager is a picky eater who refuses to eat the variety of foods we recommend, no matter how attractively they're cooked and served, I suggest that you take this matter up with his physician. If the doctor suspects that your child is not getting enough iron in his diet, a vitamin supplement with iron might be the answer.

KICKING THE SUGAR AND SALT HABITS

Your efforts to limit the sugar in your school-ager's diet should be focused on the foods he eats at home. Obviously that means that high-sugar, high-calorie, low nutrition desserts must cease to be the pièce de résistance at the end of family meals. The Eden diet recommends that you serve fresh fruit instead. I am not suggesting that cake or pie never should appear on the table, only that cake or pie should be considered special treats to be served on special occasions only.

Between-meal snacks, which supply over 30 percent of the total calories of the typical American diet, are a major source of sugar for the school-ager. If you're concerned about good nutrition, you can't have him eating unlimited junk-food snacks. Take a few minutes to go through your house and clear out the cookies and the little plastic-wrapped cakes. Get rid of the soda pop and the high-sugar instant drink mixes. Once they're gone, resolve firmly not to buy any more. Think of it this way: If these undesirable foods are not on your kitchen shelves or in the refrigerator, your school-ager can't eat them—at least not when he's at home. Replace the bad stuff with the good stuff: yogurt, cheese, fruit, crunchy raw vegetables, whole-grain bread and cereal products, low-fat milk. And make sure these wholesome foods are always within reach.

You cannot control what your child eats when he is visiting friends, nor can you be absolutely sure that he won't spend his allowance on the high-sugar treats that are bad for his teeth and add unnecessary empty calories to his diet. But you *can* make it clear that you don't want him to eat too many of these things, and explain why. (Tailor your explanations to your child's age and level of comprehension, of course, and speak calmly, without nagging or accusing.)

"Less is better" should also be your motto with salt.

Even if your child has been raised on a high-salt diet up to now, he will still benefit if you get busy and make some changes.

I advise taking the following three simple steps:

1. Use little or no salt during cooking, but use other seasonings instead such as pepper and natural herbs and spices.
2. Remove the salt shaker from the table.
3. Avoid buying and serving foods that are high in salt.

As with sugar, it is impossible to control the amount of salt your school-ager gets when he is away from home. Potato chips and other salty snacks are great favorites with many children of this age, ranking second only to sweets. You can't monitor every mouthful the way you could when your child was younger, but you certainly can reason with the school-ager and can give him some basic nutritional information and hope that it makes an impression. If it does, score one for the cause of better health. If it does not, the changes you make in his diet will insure that he is at least getting less salt at home.

SCHOOL-AGE DIET GUIDELINES

The standard American diet is conspicuous for its excesses. Problems tend to arise out of eating too much of the bad things—fat, cholesterol, sugar, and salt. That is why I urge you to focus your efforts on giving your school-age child less of these bad things, rather than trying to get him to eat more of the good things. Naturally, it would be wonderful if he ate *all* the recommended foods in the suggested amounts, but this really is not necessary and you should not try to force him. Just continue to offer a wide variety of foods and even if he only eats a few mouthfuls, don't worry about it. It may take a number of months but sooner or later he will get used to eating the nutritious foods that you offer. The Eden diet provides the best possible nutrition for your school-age child—high in vitamins, iron, fiber, and all the other important nutrients children of this age range must have for continued healthy development, but lower in the fat, cholesterol, salt, and refined sugar that contribute to major health problems.

In tailoring your child's diet to these good eating principles, you will be enhancing his present well-being and development whereas at the same time making it less likely that he will develop iron deficiency or become fat. At the same time, you will be establishing the good habits that will help protect him as an adult from heart attack, stroke, hypertension, and certain cancers. Because your school-ager does not live in a vacuum, modifying his diet will of necessity mean modifying your own diet as well. You too will be eating less fat, cholesterol, salt, and refined sugar and more iron, fiber, and vitamins. That means better health for *you* also.

HEALTHY SNACKS FOR SCHOOL-AGERS

Here is a list of healthy nutritious snacks that can be offered to your school-ager between meals:

Fruits
Frozen bananas—chunks
Strawberries
Pineapple chunks
Applesauce—no sugar
Apple slices
Grapes (frozen also)
Melon balls
Raisins

Drinks
Apple juice
Apple-cranberry juice (unsweetened)
Grape juice (unsweetened)
Orange juice
Banana-skim milkshake
Strawberry yogurt shake

Cake & Cookies and Breads
Animal crackers
Sugar wafers
Blueberry-bran muffins
Bread with apple butter
Bread with peanut butter
Popcorn
Raisin bread with cream cheese
Cheese slice melted on whole-wheat bread

Vegetables
Carrot sticks
Pea pods
Celery sticks

Miscellaneous
Ice-milk
Sherbet
Frozen yogurt
Jell-O
Puddings with low-fat milk

MEAL PLANS FOR SCHOOL-AGERS

The following are one week of daily meal plans for the normal-weight school-ager.

MONDAY

BREAKFAST	1 cup fruit salad Low-fat vanilla yogurt 2 Tbs. wheat germ 1 cup apple juice

LUNCH	Roast beef sandwich with
	    4 oz. lean roast beef
	    2 slices pumpernickel bread
	    Lettuce, tomato
	    Catsup, mustard
	    1 tsp. low-fat mayonnaise
	2 graham crackers
	2 tsp. jam
	1 cup low-fat milk

DINNER	Tofu (soybean curd) 4 oz. marinated in
	    1 Tb. soy sauce mixed with garlic,
	    onions, ginger, and sugar (1 tsp.)
	    Sautéed in 2 tsp. peanut oil with green
	    and red pepper slices
	½ cup glazed carrots
	½ cup brown rice
	1 cup orange juice

SNACK CHOICES	Melted cheese (1 oz.) on 1 slice whole-wheat bread 1 cup strawberry ice-milk with ½ cup sliced strawberries 2 oatmeal cookies

TUESDAY

BREAKFAST
1 bagel with
   2 Tbs. cream cheese
1 cup orange juice

LUNCH
1 cup split pea soup
1 cup green salad with
   2 oz. sliced turkey breast
   2 oz. Swiss cheese
   2 Tbs. low-fat salad dressing
Whole-wheat roll
1 tsp. soft margarine
1 pear, sliced

DINNER
Barbecued chicken (skin removed)—1 breast or 2 thighs
½ cup carrot cole slaw made with low-fat mayonnaise—1 Tb.
½ Tb. baked potato with sour cream blended with ½ Tb. plain yogurt
1 ear corn on the cob
1 tsp. soft margarine

SNACK CHOICES
1 cup low-fat milk
4 graham crackers
1 tsp. preserves
½ cup rice pudding with raisins
1 cup low-fat milk
1 cup pineapple wedges

WEDNESDAY

BREAKFAST
1 raisin-bran muffin with
   1 tsp. peanut butter
1 cup low-fat milk

LUNCH	1 cup cooked noodles mixed with ½ cup low-fat cottage cheese 1 apple, sliced and sprinkled with Cinnamon and lemon juice 1 pumpernickel-raisin roll
DINNER	1 slice pizza Tossed salad with 1 Tb. Italian dressing Grape soda made with ⅔ cup grape juice ⅓ cup seltzer 1 cup ice-milk, topped with ½ cup blueberries
SNACK CHOICES	1 banana, mashed with 2 Tbs. sour cream ½ cup rice pudding

THURSDAY

BREAKFAST	2 scrambled eggs made with 2 egg whites, one yolk ½ oz. American cheese 2 slices whole-wheat toast with 2 tsp. margarine 1 orange 1 cup low-fat milk
LUNCH	Cream cheese and jam sandwich 2 slices raisin bread with 2 Tbs. cream cheese 2 tsp. unsweetened jam 1 cup low-fat milk 1 apple, sliced
DINNER	5 oz. chicken cutlet, breaded with 1 egg white and coated with 2 Tbs. whole-wheat bread crumbs

	Sauteed in 1 Tb. olive oil Baked with ¼ cup tomato sauce and ½ oz. mozzarella cheese 1 cup cooked noodles with 1 tsp. margarine ½ cup string breans 1 whole-wheat roll 1 frozen yogurt pop
SNACK CHOICES	1 banana, dunked in orange juice and 1 Tb. wheat germ

FRIDAY

BREAKFAST	1 cup Cheerios 1 cup low-fat milk 1 sliced banana ½ cup low-fat cocoa
LUNCH	1 cup brown rice mixed with ⅓ cup ricotta cheese ⅓ cup sliced zucchini 1 cup tomato soup made with low-fat milk 15 frozen grapes 1 cup low-fat milk
DINNER	1 3-oz. pork chop with ½ cup applesauce ½ cup mashed potatoes with 1 tsp. margarine ½ cup string beans 1 cup apple juice 1 whole-wheat fig cookie
SNACK CHOICES	1 small raisin-bran muffin 1 small whole-wheat pita bread with 1 tsp. apple butter 1 Tb. peanut butter

SATURDAY

BREAKFAST	2 frozen waffles 2 tsp. soft margarine 2 Tbs. maple syrup 1 sliced banana

LUNCH	Chicken salad sandwich made with
	    4 oz. chicken breast
	    1 Tb. mayonnaise
	    2 slices whole-wheat bread
	Celery and carrot sticks
	1 cup orange juice
	2 fig cookies

DINNER	Broiled fillet of sole (4 oz.) with
	    1 tsp. margarine
	1 cup steamed broccoli
	1 cup brown rice mixed with
	    2 Tbs. ricotta cheese
	1 cup low-fat milk
	1 orange

SNACK CHOICES	1 pita round with
	    1 Tb. peanut butter
	    ½ cup low-fat milk
	1 oz. Mozzarella cheese stick

SUNDAY

BREAKFAST	2 small pancakes served with
	    ¼ cup frozen blueberries
	    Topped with 1 Tb. maple syrup and
	    1 tsp. margarine
	1 cup orange juice

LUNCH	Tunafish sandwich made with
	    3 oz. tuna, drained
	    1 Tb. mayonnaise

	2 slices whole-wheat bread 2 carrots, cut into sticks 1 cup low-fat milk
DINNER	4 oz. lean ground beef hamburger 1 whole-wheat roll 1 Tb. catsup ½ cup oven-baked french fries ½ cup cooked spinach 1 cup low-fat milk 1 sliced apple
SNACK CHOICES	½ cup chocolate pudding made with low-fat milk 1 cup fruit-flavored yogurt

CHAPTER 13 How to Get Your Adolescent to Eat Right

A mother once remarked to me that the adolescent is "a different animal altogether." Like many parents, she was puzzled, sometimes amused, and almost totally unprepared for the rapid changes she saw taking place in her child.

And it is no wonder. Adolescence *is* a period of enormous physical and psychological changes that seem to occur almost overnight. The studious school-ager may, for example, suddenly have trouble concentrating, and even begin to question why good grades should be all-important. The usually sweet-natured child may become nasty and disagreeable. The meticulous youngster turns into a slob.

This is a time of raging hormones and rapid growth, of fears and frustrations, of selfishness on the one hand and soaring idealism on the other. But most of all, the adolescent is characterized by a strong desire for greater independence and a need to define herself vis-à-vis, you, her parents.

It is this quest for independence that is at the heart of adolescent rebellion. To illustrate, if *you*, let us say, choose the color blue, chances are your adolescent will prefer some other color, probably the one all her friends like. Now, she may not prefer the other color for the rest of her life. In fact, in a few years, she may come around to your viewpoint and agree that blue is pretty terrific after all. But for now, it is any color *but* blue for the simple reason that blue is *your* color and she needs to assert herself in order to be able to find her own identity.

What does all this have to do with the adolescent diet plan? I think you can guess. Given the need of the normal adolescent to be her own person, it is easy to see why she will either tune out, or even adopt an opposing stance when mom and dad get too preachy about good nutrition.

Thus at about the time your child's hormones start changing you will have to play a less active role in the important area of diet. You're going to have to step back a bit and sometimes even become a silent partner in this enterprise. Believe me, as a pediatrician and as the father of two splendid young adults, I know whereof I speak.

A good diet is just as important now (maybe even more important) during your child's adolescent years than when she was younger. You should still be every bit as concerned about her health. But I know from vast experience that parents who push and pressure their teen-ager meet with more resistance and ultimately achieve less than parents who *quietly* do what needs to be done.

If I were going to write a short paragraph for parents who want to give their adolescents all the important health benefits of appropriate diet, I'd say, "Offer the best possible nutrition at home, don't bring junk food into the house, set a good example, and don't nag. PERIOD."

Of course, if your teen-ager asks for evidence, give it (but I wouldn't hold my breath waiting to be asked if I were you). If compliments are in order, as with an overweight teen-ager who manages to lose a few pounds, by all means offer them. Everybody needs to have his or her self-esteem built up, including the adolescent. But otherwise, a basically "hands-off" policy in terms of policing, supervising, and lecturing is in order.

"Is it *really* possible to modify my teen-ager's diet for the better without nagging or forcing?" Many parents of adolescents have asked me this question. The answer is yes, it can be done, and it *should* be done. I won't insult your intelligence by telling you that it will be easy. By the time a child enters adolescence, food patterns are already well established and she will want to keep on eating the same way as she has in the past. But it is *never* too late to make changes.

As long as your child lives at home and *you* plan and prepare the family meals, there will be opportunities to improve her diet. Seize these opportunities and you will help insure better health for her now and in the future.

TYPICAL ADOLESCENT NUTRITION

"I swear, my boy doesn't chew his food, he inhales it!" "He's practically eating us out of house and home!" I have heard these words or others similar from literally hundreds of parents of adolescents. Mothers and fathers are awestruck by the sheer amount of food their youngsters are suddenly capable of consuming. There's no mystery about the enormous increase in appetite that occurs sometimes during adolescence which, remember, is a time of extremely rapid growth. (Teen-agers can shoot up two or three inches in a matter of months.) Children this age tend to eat more, a *lot* more in many instances, simply because they need more food to fuel the rapid adolescent growth spurt.

Thus increased appetite leading to increased food consumption is characteristic of adolescent eating patterns. Except when a teen-ager is obese, eating large amounts of food in itself is no cause for alarm. It is *what* the adolescent eats that is worrisome. If her diet is loaded with fat and cholesterol, sugar and salt, but deficient in fiber, iron, and other essential nutrients, she is headed for trouble. Unfortunately, such a diet is pretty standard for most Americans, adolescents included. As a matter of fact, teen-agers are among the very worst nourished groups of our population.

Here, for example, is a day's worth of food as reported to me by one of my honest teen-age patients:

7:00 A.M.
- Plain donut and cup of coffee

8:15 A.M. (on way to school)
Small bag of potato chips

12:00 NOON
Pizza, cola, and chocolate ice cream cone

3:30 P.M. (on way home)
French fries and orange drink

4:30 P.M.
Cream-filled chocolate cookies and glass of milk

6:30 P.M.
Spaghetti with meat sauce (three helpings)
Bread and butter
Sliced tomatoes
Piece of apple pie
Fruit punch

9:30 P.M. (out with friends)
Vanilla ice cream cone
Hot dog on a roll
Soda

11:00 P.M.
Chocolate chip cookies

It is a nutritionist's nightmare! Although the spaghetti with meat sauce, the bread, the sliced tomatoes, pizza, and roll are all nourishing foods, almost all other items on this menu are junk, offering little other than fat, sugar or salt, and calories. I asked this same sixteen year old whether her food intake that day was typical. She shrugged and said that, yes, it was, more or less. In talking with other teen-agers, I find that on any given day their diets are likely to be similar to this young woman's. Fruits and vegetables are conspicuous by their absence, whereas foods high in fat, sugar and salt predominate.

WHAT YOU CAN DO

How can you as a parent alter the nutritional balance of your adolescent's diet in favor of more health-enhancing fruits, vegetables, fish, lean meats, and whole-grain foods? How can you help your child eat less of the high-fat, high-sugar, high-salt foods?

Let's begin with breakfast, the first meal of the day, and if not *the* most important meal, at least *as* important as the others. Too important, in fact, to be left to chance! There's only one way to make sure that your adolescent gets a good breakfast, and that is to prepare and serve it yourself! I can almost hear the groans from parents who have turned over the responsibility for making breakfast to their teen-ager. It is much easier to let her fix her own breakfast. For one thing, it allows you to get a few extra minutes of needed sleep in the morning. For another, you postpone the first argument of the day with your testy teen-ager. But if you're really serious about better nutrition, you are just going to have to set the alarm clock to go off fifteen or twenty minutes earlier and use the time to put good food on the table. If the food is ready when your teen-ager is rushing to get ready for school there is a much better chance that she will take the few minutes necessary to eat the breakfast you prepared.

A good nutritious breakfast need not be elaborate nor does it necessarily require cooking. For example, hot or cold cereal, preferably iron fortified (but not the presweetened kind) makes an excellent breakfast main course. You can add extra nutritional benefits and make the cereal more appealing by topping it with sliced strawberries, a banana, peach, or other fruit. Milk should be low-fat or skimmed. A slice of whole-grain toast plus a serving of a citrus fruit or juice completes the meal. No big deal, but if you expect your teen-ager to prepare and serve himself that type of breakfast, forget it.

There is a world of nutritional difference between the Eden breakfast I have just described and the sweet roll and coffee that so many teen-agers eat on the run. Our breakfast supplies fiber-rich whole grains, protein, calcium, and vitamins; the teen-agers' usual breakfast offers practically nothing except fat, sugar, and calories. By getting up a little earlier and offering your adolescent a well-balanced breakfast, you can add immeasurably to the nutritional content of her daily diet.

Some parents are skeptical when I urge them to supervise breakfast. "My Terry would *never* eat all that stuff," one mother exclaimed. But a few weeks later she admitted to being wrong, because Terry, it turned out, ate every bite of the new improved breakfast. As an added bonus, these short sit-down breakfasts together allowed mother and daughter to communicate with each other much more effectively than in the past.

By adolescence, many formerly picky eaters become less finicky about food. As one amazed father said to me, "There was a time when our daughter, Joan, only ate hamburgers. Now she will eat practically anything that doesn't jump off the plate." Like most human beings, however, teen-agers are inclined to do what comes easiest. Given a choice between preparing their own well-balanced breakfast and grabbing a pastry, most will go for the pastry every time. It simply isn't enough to instruct your child on the subject of a well-balanced breakfast and then expect her to prepare her own meals following your guidelines. Though a few very responsive, mature adolescents might go along with their parents' wishes on this score, my experience tells me that compliance is relatively rare and usually short-lived. In the vast majority of households the only way to make sure a teen-ager gets a good breakfast is for a parent (it doesn't always have to be mother) to prepare and serve it. Now it's dad's turn to groan.

The same is true for lunch. Of course, the days when kids came home from school for the midday meal are pretty well over. Parents can do the next-best thing, however, and pack a good nutritious lunch. Fixing a brown bag lunch for your teen-ager is usually preferable to giving her the money to pay for food in the school cafeteria or local coffee shop, for the simple reason that this gives you a greater degree of control over what she eats. Further, many school lunch programs still leave a lot to be desired when it comes to proper nutrition.

Like breakfast, lunch can be highly nutritious yet simple and easy to prepare. Sandwiches are fine if the filling is lean meat, chicken or tunafish, low-fat cheese, peanut butter, or an occasional egg. Whole-grain bread is preferable to plain white. Round out lunch with low-fat or skim milk, raw vegetables, and a piece of fruit for dessert. There is no reason to include candy, cake, soft drinks, or chips. Your teen-ager, if she is typical, probably buys far too many of these high-sugar or high-fat "nonfoods" for herself. There is no way to prevent her from doing so. The last thing you want to do is encourage her to eat more of this junk by slipping it into her lunch box.

Of course, if your child has been eating lunch in school, the switch to a brown bag lunch will mean some more extra work for you. *You* will have to assemble and pack the meal for the same reason that you must be responsible for preparing breakfast: It's the only way that you can know for sure that your child will have good nutritious food at lunchtime. If she refuses to take the lunch with her, don't fight or argue about it. Let it go for now.

Dinner is the easiest meal of all. By preparing the specific meal plans at the end of this chapter, you will be serving your entire family a diet that is low in fat and cholesterol, low in sugar and salt, and high in iron, fiber, and other important nutrients.

Earlier, I emphasized the futility of nagging your youngster about the food she eats. It is inappropriate and counterproductive. However, I believe it is entirely appropriate and productive to insist that your teen-ager be present at the evening meal. If at all possible, try serving dinner at the same time each night and let your child know that you expect her to eat with the family, not just occasionally but every single day. Once you have got her to the table, don't pressure her about eating. Let her decide how much or how little of the various items on the menu she wants.

And there you have it—the Eden diet plan for making sure your adolescent gets a well-balanced, nutritionally sound diet each day. If you prepare a well-balanced breakfast, send a healthy brown bag lunch along with her to school, cook nutritious dinners, and insist that she sit down with the rest of the family, you can be assured that your child will get enough of all the good things she needs for robust health and development during this important stage of her life. In fact, if all she ever ate was the diet we advocate and encourage, her future risk for obesity, high blood pressure, and heart problems would be significantly reduced.

TEENAGE SNACK ATTACKS

But as every parent of a teen-ager knows, they are very big on snacking and unfortunately high fat, high sugar, high-salt junk foods are the snacks of choice. You can do your bit to encourage healthier between-meal eating by not buying and bringing home the bad stuff. That means keeping the potato chips, cookies, cakes, soda pop, and sweetened drink mixes out of the house and thus out of reach of your adolescent, at least while she is at home. Instead stock up on yogurt, low-fat cheese, vegetables that can be eaten raw, fruits, and unsweetened fruit juices. Further along in this chapter is an extensive healthy snack list that you can choose from.

As for the food your child eats away from home, I'm afraid there is no way to influence what she eats on the way to and from school, at parties, on dates, after the movies, or when she goes out with friends. In fact, it is probably wise for you to assume the worst. Some teen-agers live almost entirely on fast-foods. Many parents become discouraged when they confront the fact that though their children are eating well at home, they're eating very poorly indeed when they're out of the house. These parents often wonder if it is worth bothering about, cooking and preparing good healthy meals when their youngsters eat so much unhealthy food when they're out with friends.

Believe me, I understand the frustration. It is obvious, however, that good nutrition *most* or some of the time is healthier than poor nutrition *all* of the time. In other words, your child will be much better off eating at least one healthy meal a day at home plus junk foods and fast-foods than she would be if you provided no nutritious meals at all. If your adolescent is eating the bad stuff away from home (as most kids do), it's even more important that you offer the best possible nutrition at family meals. Setting the example at home with proper nutrition is an absolute must if your goal is to protect your teen-ager from the common, dangerous food-linked health problems that afflict so many in our population.

THE ADOLESCENT AND THE CASE AGAINST FAT AND CHOLESTEROL

A high saturated-fat, high cholesterol diet makes heart attacks more likely. Of course, heart attacks are rare among teen-agers, but it may surprise you to learn that in some teen-agers the stage is already set for future catastrophe. We know this because of evidence that turned up by autopsies performed on American G.I.'s who died in Korea and Vietnam. Many of these young men, in their late teens and early twenties, from communities and cities all across the United States, already had an alarming amount of the fatty material called plaque in their arteries.

When does plaque cause problems? When arteries to the heart become sufficiently clogged with this substance, consisting mainly of cholesterol, the flow of blood is interrupted and the result is a heart attack. Similarly, heavy plaque build-up in the arteries leading to the brain can cause a stroke.

How did all that plaque form in the arteries of our young soldiers? The evidence points to the diet as the main culprit—specifically the high saturated-fat, high cholesterol diet that is so common in the United States today. We know that this type of diet is linked closely to high levels of cholesterol in the blood.

Equally telling is the fact that autopsies done on young Korean and Vietnamese soldiers, whose traditional diet of rice, vegetables, and fish is very low in saturated fat and cholesterol, showed little or no arterial plaque.

Further reenforcing the case is the heart attack and mortality rate of the United States versus Japan: Ours is several times higher; however, as the Japanese have begun to adopt a more westernized eating style with more meat and deli products, their incidence of heart attack has started to increase.

The more we learn the clearer it becomes that all the good tasting beef, the plentiful pork and lamb, the affordable whole milk and eggs and hard cheeses that we Americans look on as essential to our good health and the good health of our children actually put all of us at greater risk for heart attack and other medical disasters.

Epidemiological studies done with American-Japanese population groups also supply important evidence for a food/cancer link. For example, the incidence of breast and colon cancer in our population as a whole is quite high, but is much lower in groups such as the Seventh Day Adventists, who practice vegetarianism and use much less fat and cholesterol in their diets than other Americans. The Japanese, with their traditional low-fat, low-cholesterol, rice-vegetable-fish diet, also have a low rate of breast and colon cancer. The incidence of those cancers is higher among Japanese immigrants in the United States who have adopted the standard American diet.

Some parents worry when I recommend that they serve less red meats to their adolescents. "Doesn't my son need as much protein as he possibly can get now while he's growing like a weed?" asked the mother of fifteen-year-old Russell. The answer, of course, is that growing children *do* need sufficient quantities of protein. But red meat isn't the only source of protein nor is it necessarily the best source, as this mother seemed to believe. Fish, poultry, and veal are excellent sources of protein as are low-fat milk, yogurt and cheese, peanut butter, legumes such as kidney beans, lentils, and dried peas and beans.

"Okay, Dr. Eden, you have convinced me of the importance of cutting back on fat and cholesterol, but my kid practically lives on hamburgers. It's the only food I *know* he will eat. What if he won't go along with the changes you want me to make?" This particular question from the mother of a growing adolescent boy was not too difficult to answer. Don't worry ahead of time about how your child might react to a new style of eating, I told her. Don't even discuss with him ahead of time the changes you plan to make. Your kid may turn out to be less in love with hamburgers than you think and, believe it or not, may even welcome greater variation if the new foods are attractively cooked and served.

But even if your adolescent fusses about not getting the foods she's accustomed to, don't give in. Remember, you are still in charge of family meals and you should decide what is to be served, based on what you know to be healthiest for her. One factor in your favor is the fact that during adolescence, her appetite usually is pretty hearty. If you stand firm and continue to serve more of the good things and less of the bad, she will eventually accept, benefit, and may even enjoy the new healthier style of cooking.

ADOLESCENTS STILL NEED IRON

For young adolescents the minimum daily iron requirement is 11 milligrams per day. After the onset of menstruation, the need for iron in girls rises to 18 milligrams per day. In any event, the amount of iron required for optimal health is not so great that it cannot easily be met by a diet that includes a variety of readily available foods. (A table listing of the iron-rich foods can be found on pages 35–36.)

Adolescent iron deficiency (aside from the monthly loss of iron because of menstruation) has to do with the fact that many of the iron-rich foods simply are not perceived by teen-agers to be appealing. Red meat, a good source of iron is the exception, but liver, perhaps the best iron source of all, is shunned by many, as are leafy green vegetables, dried fruits, and legumes. When I show the parents of teen-agers a list of the foods their children should eat in order to insure an adequate supply of iron, many of them throw up their hands and say, "There's no way in the world that my child will go for that stuff!" Often, a parent's judgment of what her teen-ager will and will not eat is based on what she refused when she was much younger. In other words, they assume that because their child objected to certain foods in earlier years when her appetite was small and her whole approach to eating was less enthusiastic, she will still refuse those foods as a teen-ager. As a result, the foods that she disliked at age four or five have been absent from the family table ever since. Most youngsters, however, as they grow into adolescence, become more adventurous with regard to what they eat. That, plus the fact that appetites inevitably improve during the teen years often results in a new acceptance of previously despised foods. To those parents who believe that their kids won't eat iron-rich foods I say, "You may be wrong." Run some of these items past them again and see what happens. You may be pleasantly surprised.

But if time has not modified food preferences after all and your adolescent still balks at eating the iron-rich foods we encourage in the Eden diet, just let it go at that. Kids this age are bound and determined to do certain things *their* own way and will only dig in their heels and become more stubborn when you try to force them to eat.

You must continue to offer a wide variety of iron-rich foods whether or not your teen-ager eats them. For one thing you need iron just as much as she does, and it makes no sense to deprive yourself on her account. You may be interested to know that estimates are that close to 50 percent of all women of childbearing age in the United States suffer from some degree of iron deficiency. Just as important is the possibility that your child will become accustomed to seeing these foods on the table and watching you, her parents, enjoying them. She may eventually give them a chance herself.

THE SUGAR AND SALT DILEMMA

The child who has been allowed to eat unlimited sweets since birth is often a "sugar junkie" by adolescence. Because sweets taste so good, they're irresistible to all but the most strong-willed adolescent. The result: Teen-agers fill up on high-sugar foods that are lacking in protein, vitamins, and minerals and other essential nutrients, but which add large numbers of calories to their diets. The sweets, in turn, dull the appetite for other more nutritious foods and so contribute to deficiencies in vital nutrients and minerals.

But what if sweets do not reduce a youngster's appetite for healthy foods? What if she has the capacity to overindulge in candy and cookies between meals and can still polish off a good-sized lunch and dinner? In that case, obesity, with all its negative physical and psychological implications may result.

If your teen-ager is already a sugar junkie, you won't be able to talk her out of her habit, so save your breath. But, you can reduce her sugar intake by discontinuing highly sweetened foods at family meals and by not keeping high-sugar snack foods on hand in the house. That means no more cakes and pies, no more ice cream or pudding desserts except on special occasions. No more stocking up on cookies, sugary soft drinks, and instant drink mixes.

Of course, most teen-agers have money of their own and they eat out a lot. There's not much you can do about the sweets that are eaten outside the home. Just keep in mind and be consoled by the fact that your child, if she gets very little sugar at home but buys sweets with her own money, still will be getting less sugar than if her sugar habit were also indulged by you.

If we took a poll, we would find that there are more self-confessed sugar freaks in the United States than salt freaks (although I myself am one of the latter, preferring olives to chocolate bars any day), but many people who consider themselves indifferent to the taste of salt almost certainly still eat more of it than is consistent with good nutrition. This is true partly because salt is a hidden ingredient in many processed foods and partly because so much salt is used routinely in cooking and from the salt shaker during mealtimes.

I worry (and I hope you worry as well) about a high salt intake because of its relationship to hypertension. High blood pressure is dangerous because of its relationship to strokes, heart attacks, and kidney problems.

It would be misleading to state that a high salt diet *causes* high blood pressure, because we simply have not nailed down the evidence to prove it. But we do know that in populations where the salt intake is high, as it is here in the United States, the incidence of hypertension is also high. On the other hand, in societies that eat less salt, high blood pressure is rare. It has also been demonstrated that a reduction in dietary salt results in the lowering of blood pressure. In fact, as you probably know, a salt-restricted diet is a mandatory part of treatment of hypertension. Evidence certainly tends to incriminate a high salt diet as a factor in the development of hypertension.

Hypertension, contrary to what many people believe, is not limited to adults. We are now finding high blood pressure in pre-schoolers, school-age children, and adolescents. During the teen-age years the incidence of high blood pressure is approximately 5 percent and even higher in black teen-agers. In the adult population one out of eight, or 12 percent, suffers from this condition. The obvious question is whether adult hypertension starts during childhood. I can't answer with a straight unqualified yes. However, the evidence to date has prompted a general consensus among pediatricians that the longer a child eats a diet that is too high in salt, the greater the risk for the subsequent development of high blood pressure.

One of the most important things you can do for the present and future health of your adolescent (and for everyone else in your family as well) is to limit the amount of salt consumed at home. You can cut back on in-house salt consumption by a whopping two-thirds if you simply reduce the amounts added to food during cooking, serve fewer canned, smoked, pickled, salt-cured, frozen prepared foods, and salty snack foods, and *remove* the salt shaker from the table.

As for the salty foods your adolescent eats away from home, I am sure by now you know my thoughts about that. You can't and should not police your child's diet where outside eating is concerned. Your warnings won't work and probably will become an additional source of parent-teen tension. Simply do your part at home—the salt she won't be eating there will help counterbalance the salt she may be getting elsewhere—that's the Eden Diet philosophy.

ADOLESCENT DIET GUIDELINES

The typical youngster actually doubles her body mass between the ages of ten and eighteen. To fuel this tremendous growth spurt the adolescent needs plenty of food—more in fact than at any other time in her young life!

An adequate number of calories per day is a must, of course. But equally important is that those calories be supplied by foods rich in all the nutritional elements that children of this age need for optimal growth and development. The Eden diet plan meals that follow for adolescent boys and girls are based on such nutrient-rich foods. The breakfasts, lunches, dinners, and snacks on the following pages will provide your youngster with more than enough of the protein, complex carbohydrates, vitamins, and minerals she needs during this crucial growth period, but with less of the fat, cholesterol, salt, and refined sugar that contribute to some of the most serious health problems besetting our population.

HEALTHY SNACKS FOR TEEN-AGERS

Here is a list of healthy snacks for normal-weight teen-agers.

Fruit
Pineapple wedges
Grapes (frozen too)
Cherries
Apples
Pears
Frozen bananas

Dried Fruit
Raisins
Prunes
Dates
Figs

Ice Creams/Puddings
Fudgecicle
Ice-milk—soft or hard
Italian ices
Sherbet
Frozen yogurt (soft serve)
Frozen yogurt bar
Puddings made with low-fat milk
Indian pudding
Chocolate shakes made with low-fat milk

Breads, Cereals, and Grains
Popcorn—unbuttered
Pretzels—some salt removed
Open pizza made with ½ English muffin, melted cheese, and tomato
Soups—bean, vegetable, minestrone,
chicken noodle, split pea with low-fat milk, or broth
Bread sticks
Bran cereal with low-fat milk
Bran, corn, or blueberry muffins
Pita bread with 1 Tb. peanut butter
½ bagel with 1 Tb. cream cheese
Melba toast with jam

Cakes and Cookies
Angel food cake
Sponge cake
Fig bars

Vegetables
Carrot sticks
Zucchini sticks
Celery
Tossed salad

MEAL PLANS FOR ADOLESCENTS

The meal plans that follow have been divided into four groups (each for one week) in order to accommodate the differing caloric needs of the normal weight-growing male teen-ager, fully grown male teen-ager, growing female teen-ager, and fully grown female teen-ager. (See Chapter 00 for menu plans for overweight adolescents.) These diet plans have been designed not only to fit the basic guidelines of the Eden diet, but to include foods that teen-agers enjoy.

GROWING MALE TEEN-AGER

MONDAY

BREAKFAST	1 cup orange juice ¾ cup granola 1 cup low-fat milk

LUNCH	Tunafish sandwich made with 2 slices rye bread
	   ¾ cup tuna salad with 2 Tbs. mayonnaise
	   Celery and onion, chopped
	½ cup cole slaw
	Milkshake with
	   1 cup low-fat milk
	   ½ cup ice cream

DINNER	Hamburger
	   6 oz. lean ground beef
	   1 oz. cheese
	   1 roll
	   Catsup
	1 cup string beans, steamed
	1 cup oven-baked potato wedges
	1 pat margarine
	1 grape juice

SNACK CHOICES	1 bran muffin 1 cup apple juice 1 apple

TUESDAY

BREAKFAST	2 frozen waffles with
	    2 Tbs. maple syrup
	½ cup vanilla yogurt
	    ½ cup sliced strawberries

LUNCH	1 cup lentil soup
	4 oz. sliced turkey breast on
	    1 hard roll with
	    1 Tb. Russian dressing
	    Lettuce and tomato
	1 cup apple juice

DINNER	2 slices pizza Tossed salad with 2 Tbs. salad dressing 1 cup seltzer with grape juice
SNACK CHOICES	1 small bag salt-free pretzels ⅔ cup orange sherbet made with vanilla ice-milk 1 piece carrot bread 1 cup low-fat milk

WEDNESDAY

BREAKFAST	1½ cups raisin bran with 1 cup low-fat milk ½ cantaloupe
LUNCH	1 large pita bread round, stuffed with Fresh vegetables

DIET-PLAN MENUS FOR HEALTHIER EATING

2 oz. shredded cheese
Tomato slices
1 Tb. salad dressing
1 cup apple juice

DINNER
2 cups spaghetti
¾ cup tomato sauce with
  Eggplant, mushrooms, and onions
  Sautéed in 1 Tb. olive oil
3 Tbs. Parmesan cheese
2 slices (1 oz. each) whole wheat Italian bread
  2 tsp. margarine
1 cup seltzer
1 frozen fruit bar

SNACK CHOICES
1 strawberry yogurt
1 orange
3 cups air-popped popcorn
1 cup fresh fruit salad

THURSDAY

BREAKFAST
1 cup oatmeal
1 cup low-fat milk
½ banana, sliced
½ cup orange juice

LUNCH
Tunafish sandwich
  4 oz. tuna
  1 Tb. mayonnaise
  1 hard roll
  Lettuce and tomato
Celery and carrot sticks
1 pear

DINNER
2 bean enchiladas made with
  1 cup cooked kidney or pinto beans
  2 tortillas

2 oz. shredded cheese
½ cup tomato sauce
¾ cup brown rice
Tossed salad with
   2 Tbs. dressing
1 cup apple juice

SNACK CHOICES

1 bran muffin
1 cup low-fat milk
4 graham crackers with
   4 tsp. peanut butter
1 cup frozen yogurt

FRIDAY

BREAKFAST

1 bagel
   2 Tbs. cream cheese
1 cup orange juice

LUNCH

1 cup vegetable soup
Chicken breast sandwich made with
   4 oz. sliced chicken
   2 slices rye bread
   1 Tb. mayonnaise
½ cup cole slaw
1 cup low-fat milk

DINNER

6 oz. broiled swordfish, marinated in
   Soy sauce, lemon juice, garlic, and ginger
1 cup stir-fried snow peas and mushrooms in:
1 Tb. sesame oil
1 cup brown rice
½ cantaloupe
½ cup ice-milk

SNACK CHOICES

1 cup low-fat milk
1 medium corn muffin with 1 tsp. strawberry jam
3 cups air-popped popcorn
1 cup low-fat milk

SATURDAY

BREAKFAST	2 pancakes with
	    2 Tbs. maple syrup
	    1 tsp. soft margarine
	1 cup orange juice

LUNCH	2 slices pizza 1 cup low-fat milk 1 apple

DINNER	6 oz. boneless chicken breast, stir-fried with
	    1 cup mushrooms
	    1 cup broccoli
	    ½ cup chopped onion
	    1 Tb. safflower oil
	Served on
	    1 cup thin spaghetti
	    1 cup pineapaple chunks
	½ cup grape juice, mixed with
	    ½ cup seltzer

SNACK CHOICES	½ bagel with 1 Tb. cream cheese 1 cup low-fat milk ½ cup ice-milk 1 cup vanilla pudding made with low-fat milk

SUNDAY

BREAKFAST	1 cup shredded wheat with
	    1 cup low-fat milk and
	    ½ cup blueberries
	1 cup orange juice

LUNCH	Tuna melt made with
	    4 oz. tuna
	    1 Tb. mayonnaise

	1 slice Swiss cheese
	2 tomato slices
	1 cup split pea soup
	½ cup low-fat milk
	1 orange
DINNER	Barbecued chicken made with
	2 chicken breasts
	2 Tbs. barbecue sauce mixed with
	1 Tb. apricot preserves
	1 baked potato with 1 tsp. margarine
	2 Tbs. sour cream
	1 cup steamed asparagus
	1 piece sponge cake
	1 cup low-fat milk
SNACK CHOICES	¼ cup mixed raisins and peanuts
	2 rice cakes
	½ cup cranberry juice mixed with ½ cup seltzer
	Milkshake made with ½ banana
	½ cup low-fat milk
	1 tsp. honey

GROWING FEMALE TEEN-AGER

MONDAY

BREAKFAST	½ cup orange juice
	2 pancakes with
	1 tsp. margarine
	2 Tbs. syrup
	1 cup low-fat milk
LUNCH	1 roast beef sandwich made with
	3 oz. lean roast beef
	1 Tb. catsup

	2 slices of whole-wheat bread 1 apple 1 cup low-fat milk

DINNER	Chicken Parmesan made with
	   5 oz. boneless, skinless chicken breast, browned in
	   2 tsp. olive oil
	   baked with 1 cup of tomato sauce and 2 oz. of part-skim mozzarella cheese and 1 Tb. Parmesan cheese
	Served on 1 cup noodles
	1 cup steamed broccoli
	½ cup grape juice with ½ cup seltzer

SNACK CHOICES	2 oatmeal cookies ½ cup low-fat milk 1 cup grapes

TUESDAY

BREAKFAST	1 cup oatmeal 1 orange 1 cup low-fat milk

LUNCH	Turkey sandwich
	   4 oz. turkey breast
	   2 slices pumpernickel bread
	   1 Tb. Russian dressing
	   Lettuce and tomato
	   1 pear

DINNER	2 broiled pork chops, trimmed of fat
	½ cup applesauce
	1 cup oven-baked "french fries"
	   1 Tb. catsup
	1 slice rye bread
	   1 tsp. margarine
	1 cup broccoli

	½ cup grape juice mixed with ½ cup seltzer
SNACK CHOICES	1 frozen yogurt pop 1 cup lentil soup 2 saltines—salt-free ½ bagel with 1 Tb. peanut butter

WEDNESDAY

BREAKFAST	1 cup raisin bran ½ sliced banana 1 cup low-fat milk
LUNCH	1 bagel with 2 oz. melted Swiss cheese 1 Tb. mustard 1 orange 1 cup low-fat milk
DINNER	6 oz. broiled swordfish, marinated in Soy sauce, lemon juice, garlic, and ginger 1 cup stir-fried snow peas and mushrooms 1 Tb. sesame oil 1 cup brown rice ½ cup apple juice 2 fig cookies ½ cup low-fat milk
SNACK CHOICES	1 baked apple with 2 Tbs. cottage cheese 1 cup ice-milk

THURSDAY

BREAKFAST	½ bagel with 1 Tb. cream cheese Sliced tomato ½ cup orange juice

LUNCH	4 oz. lean roast beef
	  2 slices pumpernickel bread
	  1 Tb. Russian dressing
	½ cup grape juice
	1 apple

DINNER	Macaroni and cheese
	  Mix together and bake:
	  1½ cups cooked macaroni
	  2 oz. cheese
	  ¼ cup low-fat milk
	1 pumpernickel roll
	  1 tsp. margarine
	½ cup apple juice

SNACK CHOICES	1 cup fruit salad with
	  ½ cup low-fat vanilla yogurt
	2 oatmeal cookies
	1 cup low-fat milk
	2 rice cakes with
	  2 tsp. peanut butter

FRIDAY

BREAKFAST	1 cup fortified bran flakes 1 cup low-fat milk ½ cup sliced strawberries

LUNCH	1 cup cooked noodles mixed with
	  3 oz. tunafish and
	  2 Tbs. cottage cheese
	½ cup carrots glazed with
	  1 tsp. orange marmalade
	2 oatmeal cookies
	1 cup low-fat milk

DINNER	Chicken with mustard sauce
	  4 oz. skinless chicken breast
	  Marinated in 2 Tbs. mustard and
	  1 Tb. each:

Safflower oil, soy sauce, and honey
1 cup steamed cauliflower
1 cup rice pilaf
1 cup diced pineapple

SNACK CHOICES
1 uncoated frozen yogurt pop
1 cup split pea soup
2 whole-wheat crackers
1 piece whole-wheat bread with
  1 Tb. peanut butter
  1 tsp. apple butter
1 cup low-fat milk

SATURDAY

BREAKFAST
2 slices rye toast with
  2 tsp. margarine
  1 tsp. jelly
1 scrambled egg
1 cup orange juice

LUNCH
Large tossed salad with
  3 oz. turkey breast
  1 oz. cheese
  2 Tbs. salad dressing
1 pumpernickel-raisin roll
  1 tsp. margarine
1 apple
1 cup low-fat milk

DINNER
4 oz. lean hamburger
  1 roll
  1 Tb. catsup
½ cup peas
1 baked sweet potato
  ½ Tb. each: sour cream and yogurt
½ cantaloupe
Seltzer

SNACK CHOICES	2 cups popcorn 1 cup low-fat strawberry yogurt

SUNDAY

BREAKFAST	1 poached egg 1 slice whole-wheat toast 1 tsp. jelly 1 cup orange juice

LUNCH	1 cup lentil soup with
	   2 Tbs. toasted bread cubes
	1 slice rye bread with
	   3 oz. turkey breast
	   2 Tbs. Russian dressing
	Sliced tomatoes and lettuce wedge
	1 apple

DINNER	Spaghetti with meat sauce
	   1½ cup cooked spaghetti
	   ¾ cup tomato sauce with
	   2 oz. lean chopped meat, onions, and peppers, sautéed in 1 Tb. olive oil
	   2 Tbs. Parmesan cheese
	1 slice Italian bread
	   1 tsp. margarine
	1 cup low-fat milk
	1 peach

SNACK CHOICES	½ cup chocolate pudding made with low-fat milk
	1 cup low-fat vanilla yogurt
	Banana shake made with
	   ½ cup skim milk, blended with
	   ½ banana, 2 ice cubes, and 1 tsp. honey

FULLY GROWN MALE TEEN-AGER

MONDAY

BREAKFAST
1 cup shredded wheat with
½ banana
1 cup low-fat milk
1 slice raisin bread
2 tsp. whipped cream cheese

LUNCH
1 cup chili made with kidney or pinto beans and chopped lean beef
6 saltines
1 cup apple juice

DINNER
Macaroni and cheese
2 cups of cooked macaroni with
1½ oz. American cheese
¼ cup of low-fat milk
2 cups raw vegetables with ¼ cup low-fat dip (made with low-fat mayonnaise, catsup, and relish)
1 slice Italian bread
1 tsp. margarine
1 cup orange juice

SNACK CHOICES
4 graham crackers with
1 Tb. peanut butter
½ cup low-fat milk
½ cup blueberries
½ cup low-fat vanilla yogurt

TUESDAY

BREAKFAST
2 pancakes with
3 Tbs. syrup and

152 DIET-PLAN MENUS FOR HEALTHIER EATING

                    1 tsp. margarine
                    1 cup orange juice

LUNCH   Chicken salad sandwich made with
                    5 oz. cooked chicken
                    2 Tbs. mayonnaise
                    Celery
                On a hard roll with
                    Sliced lettuce and tomato
                1 cup split pea soup
                1 cup low-fat milk

DINNER   6 oz. broiled swordfish, pan-fried in
                    1 Tb. each: sesame oil, soy sauce, lemon juice, and sesame seeds
                    Fresh garlic and ginger
                1 cup steamed broccoli
                1½ cups brown rice
                ½ cantaloupe with ½ cup ice-milk
                Seltzer

SNACK CHOICES   1 medium corn muffin with
                    1 tsp. jam
                    1 tsp. margarine
                1 cup low-fat milk
                3 cups air-popped popcorn
                1 cup cranberry-apple juice

WEDNESDAY

BREAKFAST   2 scrambled eggs
                1 banana-bran muffin with
                    2 tsp. margarine
                1 cup orange juice

LUNCH   1 cup Manhattan clam chowder
                    2 saltines
                Tunafish sandwich on a bagel with
                    4 oz. tuna

	1 Tb. mayonnaise Celery and carrots 1 cup low-fat milk 1 frozen fruit bar

DINNER	2 cups cooked spaghetti mixed with
	    2 cups assorted vegetables
	    Sautéed in 1 Tb. olive oil
	    Topped with 2 oz. part-skim mozzarella cheese
	1 slice Italian bread with
	    1 tsp. margarine
	1 cup low-fat milk

SNACK CHOICES	1 slice whole-wheat bread with 1 Tb. peanut butter 1 cup low-fat milk 1 cup low-fat lemon yogurt

THURSDAY

BREAKFAST	1 blueberry-bran muffin with
	    1 Tb. peanut butter
	    2 tsp. jelly
	1 cup low-fat milk

LUNCH	Tuna melt made with
	    4 oz. tuna
	    1 Tb. diet mayonnaise
	    2 slices pumpernickel bread
	    1 slice Swiss cheese
	    Tomato slices
	1 cup lentil soup
	1 cup low-fat milk
	1 orange

DINNER	2 slices pizza Tossed salad with 1 Tb. salad dressing

	½ cup each: seltzer and orange juice
	½ cup ice-milk
SNACK CHOICES	1 cup low-fat lemon yogurt
	1 orange
	2 whole-wheat crackers
	1 small bag salt-free pretzels

FRIDAY

BREAKFAST	1 bagel with
	2 Tbs. cream cheese
	1 Tb. jelly
	1 cup orange juice
LUNCH	2 slices pizza
	1 cup apple juice
	Tossed salad with
	2 Tbs. French dressing
DINNER	Stir-fried chicken made with
	8 oz. boneless chicken breast
	1 cup each: mushrooms and snow peas,
	½ cup onion
	Sautéed in ½ Tb. sesame oil and
	1 Tb. soy sauce
	Served on 1½ cups thin spaghetti with
	1 cup pineapple chunks
	Grape spritzer made with
	½ cup grape juice
	½ cup seltzer
SNACK CHOICES	3 dried figs
	Strawberry shake made with
	½ cup sliced strawberries
	½ cup low-fat milk
	1 cup low-fat frozen yogurt with
	sliced banana

SATURDAY

BREAKFAST	1 cup whole-grain cereal 1 banana 1 cup low-fat milk 1 slice whole-wheat bread with 1 Tb. peanut butter
LUNCH	4 oz. hamburger 1 roll 1 Tb. catsup 1 cup apple juice fresh cherries

DINNER	1½ cup vegetarian chili made with
	  1 cup cooked kidney or pinto beans
	  1 cup diced onions, peppers, and carrots
	  1 cup whole tomatoes
	  Sautéed in 1 Tb. safflower oil
	  Served on 1½ cups brown rice
	  Sprinkled with 2 Tbs. shredded cheddar cheese
	Tossed salad with
	  2 Tbs. creamy Italian salad dressing
	Orange spritzer made with
	  ½ cup each: orange juice and seltzer

SNACK CHOICES	1 piece angel food cake ½ cup low-fat milk 1 small blueberry muffin with 1 tsp. margarine 1 cup low-fat raspberry yogurt

SUNDAY

BREAKFAST	2 frozen waffles with 2 tsp. margarine

	2 Tbs. syrup ½ cup orange juice
LUNCH	2 slices pizza ½ cup grape juice Tossed salad with 2 Tbs. dressing

DINNER	6 oz. fillet of sole stuffed with
	   ½ cup spinach and
	   1 oz. feta cheese
	Baked with 1 tsp. margarine
	1 large baked sweet potato
	1 cup steamed broccoli
	2 oatmeal cookies
	1 cup low-fat milk

SNACK CHOICES	1 cup low-fat blueberry yogurt with
	   1 banana, sliced
	1 cup vanilla ice-milk with
	   ½ cup sliced strawberries

FULLY GROWN FEMALE TEEN-AGER

MONDAY

BREAKFAST	Scrambled eggs made with 1 whole egg and 1 egg white and 1 oz. cheese 1 slice rye bread 1 tsp. margarine 1 tsp. jam ½ cup orange juice

LUNCH	1 chicken salad sandwich with
	   3 oz. baked chicken breast (skinless)
	   1 Tb. low-fat mayonnaise
	   2 slices pumpernickel bread
	   Lettuce and tomato

	1 pear 1 cup apple juice
DINNER	5 oz. baked fillet of sole with garlic and 1 tsp. margarine ½ cup cole slaw 1 cup brown rice with scallions 1 cup low-fat milk
SNACK CHOICES	1 cup frozen yogurt 2 fig bars 1 cup low-fat milk

TUESDAY

BREAKFAST	½ bagel with
	   1 Tb. cream cheese
	   Sliced tomato
	½ cup orange juice

LUNCH	Chef salad made with
	   3 cups lettuce, tomato, cucumber, carrots, and cabbage
	   2 oz. turkey breast
	   1 oz. Swiss cheese
	   2 Tbs. Russian dressing
	1 pumpernickel-raisin roll
	Grape soda made with ½ cup grape juice and ½ cup seltzer

DINNER	Macaroni and cheese
	   Mix together and bake:
	   1½ cups cooked macaroni
	   2 oz. shredded cheese, and
	   ¼ cup low-fat milk
	Carrot and tomato slices
	1 slice whole-wheat bread
	1 tsp. margarine
	4 stewed prunes
	½ cup apple juice

SNACK CHOICES	1 frozen yogurt pop
	Banana shake made with
	  ½ banana
	  ½ cup low-fat milk
	1 fig bar
	½ cup low-fat milk

WEDNESDAY

BREAKFAST	1 cup whole-grain cereal 1 cup low-fat milk 1 orange

LUNCH	Turkey sandwich
	  3 oz. turkey breast
	  2 slices pumpernickel bread
	  1 Tb. Russian dressing
	  Lettuce and tomato

DINNER	2 broiled pork chops, trimmed of fat ½ cup applesauce 1 cup brown rice 1 slice whole-wheat bread 1 tsp. margarine 1 cup Brussels sprouts ½ cup grapejuice mixed with ½ cup seltzer
SNACK CHOICES	1 frozen yogurt pop 1 slice rye bread with 1 Tb. peanut butter Banana bread ½ cup low-fat milk

THURSDAY

BREAKFAST	1 cup oatmeal made with

	1 cup low-fat milk 3 Tbs. raisins
LUNCH	1 slice pizza Tossed salad with 1 Tb. Italian dressing 1 orange

DINNER	Chinese style chicken
	   Stir-fry in wok:
	   4 oz. chicken
	   ½ cup mushrooms
	   1 Tb. soy sauce
	   1 Tb. hoisin sauce
	   1 Tb. sesame oil
	Served on 1 cup cooked thin spaghetti
	Grape float, made with
	   ½ cup grape juice
	   ½ cup ice-milk

SNACK CHOICES	1 baked apple 1 slice raisin bread with 1 Tb. cream cheese Carrot bread ½ cup low-fat milk

FRIDAY

BREAKFAST	1 cup Wheaties cereal ½ banana 1 cup low-fat milk
LUNCH	1 slice pizza Tossed salad with 1 Tb. dressing ½ cup grape juice

DINNER	6 oz. broiled swordfish, marinated in
	   Soy sauce, lemon juice, garlic, ginger,
	   and 1 Tb. sesame oil

	1 cup brown rice 1 cup stir-fried asparagus ½ cup apple juice
SNACK CHOICES	2 whole-wheat fig bars 1 cup low-fat milk ½ cup ice-milk with sliced strawberries 1 baked apple

SATURDAY

BREAKFAST	1 scrambled egg
	2 slices pumpernickel toast
	  2 tsp. margarine
	  1 tsp. jelly
	½ cup orange juice

LUNCH	Tunafish sandwich
	  2 slices rye bread with
	  4 oz. tuna
	  1 Tb. low-fat mayonnaise
	  Sliced tomato and lettuce
	1 cup low-fat milk
	1 slice watermelon

DINNER	4 oz. lean hamburger
	1 whole-wheat roll
	  1 Tb. catsup
	1 small baked potato with
	  1 Tb. sour cream
	½ cup peas
	½ cantaloupe

SNACK CHOICES	2 cups air-popped popcorn 1 cup low-fat lemon yogurt

SUNDAY

BREAKFAST
1 baked appled with
   ½ cup low-fat vanilla yogurt
   1 Tb. wheat germ
½ cup unsweetened grape juice

LUNCH
Bagel with
   2 Tbs. cream cheese and
   1 Tb. jelly
½ cup low-fat milk

DINNER
1 cup spaghetti topped with
   3 oz. tofu and
   1 cup broccoli
Stir-fried in
   1 Tb. sesame oil and
   1 Tb. soy sauce
Sliced carrots and zucchini
½ cup low-fat milk
1 slice whole-wheat bread with
   1 tsp. margarine
1 pear

SNACK CHOICES
1 slice whole-wheat bread with
   1 oz. melted cheese and
   sliced tomatoes
½ cup apple juice
1 small piece angel food cake
½ cup low-fat milk

PART III
EXERCISE THAT'S FUN AND EASY

CHAPTER 14
Infant Games

The earlier an infant is started on the Eden exercise plan, the better. New babies are quite sturdy and remarkably well engineered. Despite what you may think they are not at all fragile. There is no reason for you to be afraid of handling her and moving her around, starting on day 1. The main precaution during the first month or two is to support her head, because it's still quite wobbly. Just as soon as you get home from the hospital with your new baby you can start to help her develop strength, agility, and good muscle tone.

The following are some specific infant exercise suggestions:

0–3 months

1. *Carry her around in different positions*: Infants are usually carried around in the so-called burping position up on your shoulder. By changing your carrying position you help strengthen her large muscles. An infant seat or pack sack can be used for this purpose. She can be positioned face forward or face backward.

2. *Strengthening neck muscles*: These exercises help the infant achieve better head control. Place your baby on her stomach a number of times each day. This allows her the opportunity to learn to lift her head.

3. *Leg exercises*: When lying on her back her legs can be

exercised by pumping them gently as if she were riding a bicycle.

4. *Crib devices*: This can be useful in stimulating physical activity. One example is a cradle gym; it has rings and bells attached and is hung over the crib. Most babies will start to swipe and reach at about two to three months of age, and this device gives her an excellent opportunity to exercise her arms.

There is no question that babies enjoy being handled and bounced up and down. The earlier you start, the stronger and more agile she will become. A flabby, inactive infant, even at two or three months of age, is not as healthy as a toned-up active one.

3–6 months

Three to six-month-old babies love to exercise. My best advice is to give her the space and opportunity to do so. No special equipment is necessary.

1. *Crib devices*: Your baby is learning to grasp and reach and is becoming increasingly skillful at these activities. During these months she will make excellent use of the devices attached to the crib, and this is a useful form of physical activity.

2. *Turn-over games*: Not only is this activity great fun for the baby but it is a splendid exercise as well. It tones up her muscles and increases her agility. Babies never seem to get tired of turning over again and again and again.

3. *Kicking toys*: Large cuddly kicking toys can be attached to the sides of the crib. Your infant will enjoy kicking at them and grabbing for them. Besides helping her develop leg strength, they also will keep her happy and busy.

4. *Creeping and rocking*: Five to six-month-old babies start to creep or push themselves along, either backward or forward. I recommend that you take your baby out of the crib a number of times each day, putting her on the floor or in a playpen so that she can have the space to practice these new skills.

5. *Standing*: Between three and six months of age most babies can support their weight while standing supported. It is a

good idea to get your baby on her feet, because this will help develop her leg strength and improve her large-muscle coordination. (Let me assure you that there is no truth to the old wives' tale that standing a baby up early will cause bowlegs.)

The infant who is kept swaddled and restricted, not allowed to learn to explore the environment, and not encouraged to exercise, will quickly become inactive and sedentary. If the goal is optimal physical development, you must encourage your baby to use all her muscles now.

There are a number of structured exercise programs for infants, starting at three months of age, that are mushrooming all over the country. Gymboree and Play-Arena are two examples. If one of these programs is available in your community, it might be a good idea to check it out. It not only will help get your baby moving in a happy, safe environment, but it will give you a chance to get out and meet other parents who have infants the same age as your own.

The following singing games—and other games in this chapter—are from Gymboree. Try them. You will easily see why children enjoy such programs.

Gymboree® Boogies

ROLY POLY
(Tune: "Open, Shut Them")

Position: Baby is lying on back facing parent.

Words	Movements
Roly poly, roly poly,	Rotate arms in front of chest.
Out, out, out.	Extend arms out.
Roly poly, roly poly,	Rotate arms in front of chest.
In, in, in.	Alternately cross arms.
Roly poly, roly poly,	Rotate arms in front of chest.
Touch your nose.	Touch nose.
Roly poly, roly poly,	Rotate arms in front of chest.
Touch your toes.	Pull to a sit and touch toes.

EXERCISE THAT'S FUN AND EASY

Roly poly, roly poly,	Rotate arms in front of chest.
To the sky.	Stretch arms up, pull to stand.
Roly poly, roly poly,	Rotate arms in front of chest.
Fly, fly, fly.	Lift and gently swing.

BLUE BELLS
(Chant)

Position: Baby is lying on back facing parent.

Words   *Movements*

Blue bells,   Flex knees alternately.
Cockle shells.
Eevy, ivy, over.   Flex knee while turning baby over on to his stomach.

Variations: Use this boogie with crawlers in the following manner:

Words   *Movements*

Blue bells,   Sway baby's legs side to side.
Cockle shells.
Eevy, ivy, over.   Grasp baby's ankle with one hand while placing other hand on baby's tummy. Sommersault baby, landing him on his feet or in a seated position.

WHEELS ON THE BUS
(Tune: "Wheels on The Bus")

Position: Baby is lying on back facing parent or sitting in parent's lap.

Words   *Movements*

The wheels on the bus   Rotate baby's arms in front of chest.
Go round and round.
Round and round.
Round and round.
The wheels on the bus
Go round and round.
All through the town.   Make circle with baby's arms.

2. The doors on the bus go open and shut . . .	Baby's arms go out to sides and back in.
3. The wipers on the bus go swish, swish, swish . . .	Arms together, go side to side.
4. The horn on the bus goes beep, beep, beep . . .	Touch toes to nose.

LOVE IS A CIRCLE
(Chant)

Position: Baby is lying on back facing parent.

Words	Movements
Love is a circle, Round and round.	Move baby's arms in a circular motion starting above head and crossing the front of body.
Love is up, Love is down. Love is up, Love is down.	Stretch hands up, lower.
Love is inside Trying to get out.	Knead baby's hands on stomach then stretch out to sides.
Love is whirling And twirling about.	Rotate arms in front of body.
Love is a circle Round and round.	Repeat circular motion, opposite direction.
Love in the corners Of squares can be found.	Trace a square on baby's tummy.
Love is reaching and Spreading its wings.	Pull baby to sit. Spread arms out to sides.
Love will dance	Lift baby to stand.
And love will sing!	Hold hips and sway.

TURN, TURN, TURN AROUND

Position: Baby is lying or seated facing parent.

Words	Midline
Turn, turn, turn around, Turn, turn, turn around.	Rotate baby's arms in front of chest
Up, down,	Extend baby's arms up over head, then down.
Clap, clap, clap.	Clap baby's hands.
2. Turn, turn, turn around . . . In, out . . .	Cross baby's arms across chest, then back out.
3. Turn, turn, turn around . . . Touch your nose . . .	Touch baby's nose with her hands.
4. (Touch toes, flex wrists, ankles, etc.)	

6–9 months

Between six and nine months your baby will make large advances in her physical development. She should be able to sit well, begin to stand by pulling herself up to a standing position, crawl and creep, and may even begin to "cruise" along the furniture. She will now probably be able to turn efficiently, both from front to back and back to front, and will be able to pull herself along the ground on her hands and knees. It still isn't necessary to purchase any special exercise equipment. What your baby needs is the *space* to move around—to crawl, creep, swing around, rock along, and cruise. She is eager to explore her world and needs little encouragement to move around. What she requires from you is the freedom and the opportunity to do so. There is one exception to this, and that is the baby who already is too fat. The very obese six to nine month old often is content to merely sit or lie around, preferably with a bottle of milk or juice to keep her occupied. A vicious cycle now begins. The fatter the baby the less active she becomes; the less active she is, the fewer calories she burns up, and this results in her becoming even fatter. This inactive fat baby requires extra effort on your part to encourage her to exercise in order to help break this vicious cycle.

The six to nine month old is full of life and fun and very happy to be physically handled. They love to be swung in the air, bounced up and down, and are in heaven when their mother or father gets down on the floor with them for some tussling and crawling and chasing. Promoting and encouraging physical activity at this early age will make it much more likely that she will continue to practice and enjoy physical exercise throughout her childhood and beyond. Here's more for six-to-nine-month-olds from **Gymboree®**:

JUST LIKE ME

(Tune: "London Bridges")

Position: Baby is lying on back facing parent.

Words	*Movements*
Make your arms go Up and down Up and down, up and down. Make your arms go Up and down. Just like me.	Baby does movements indicated by words.

2. Make your legs (feet, ankles, etc.)

SWAY, SWAY

(Tune: "Sway, Sway")

Position: Parent standing and holding baby under arms and away from body.

Words	*Movements*
Sway, sway, sway, sway.	Sway from side to side.
Now reach up and touch the sky.	Lift baby up over head.
Then fall gently like the snow,	Lower baby so his hands
Down to the ground.	reach out to catch himself.

X MARKS THE SPOT
(Chant)

Position: Baby is lying on tummy across parent's lap or sitting in parent's lap.

Words	*Movements*
X marks the spot,	Draw "x" across back.
With a dot and a dot,	Dot on each side of midline.
And a dash and a dash,	Dash on each side of midline.
And a big question mark.	Draw a big question mark.
With a line going up,	Hand firmly touches up,
And a line going down,	Hand touches down and
And a line going Round and round and round.	makes a circular motion.
With a hug and a squeeze,	Give baby a nice firm hug.
And a cool ocean breeze.	Blow on back of the neck.

PUSH-UPS

With an inner tube or GymTubes™ lying flat on the ground, place the infant face down so that his tummy is resting on the inflated section of the tube. Assist the infant with balance by resting your hand on the baby's bottom. Encourage him to extend his arms, so that he is supporting as much of his upper torso as possible as he raises his head. Place the mirror in front of him to encourage this behavior. As the infant becomes accustomed to supporting his weight on his arms, place a toy in front of him and encourage him to reach for it.

YEAH-YEAH
(Chant)

Position: Baby is lying on his back facing parent.

Words	*Movements*
Can you clap your feet? Yeah, Yeah.	Clap baby's feet together.

Can you clap your feet?	
Yeah, Yeah.	
Can you feel your knees?	Hold baby's knees and push
Yeah, Yeah.	up to his tummy.
Can you feel your knees?	
Yeah, Yeah.	
Can you swish your hips?	Hold baby's hips and rock
Yeah, Yeah.	side to side.
Can you swish your hips?	
Yeah, Yeah.	
Can you up and down?	Extend legs upward and
Yeah, Yeah.	then down.
Can you up and down?	
Yeah, Yeah.	
Can you clap your hands?	Clap baby's hands together.
Yeah, Yeah.	
Can you clap your hands?	
Yeah, Yeah.	
Can you feel the beat?	Clap baby's hands together.
Yeah, Yeah.	
Can you feel the beat?	
Yeah, Yeah.	
Can you side to side?	Hold baby's arms and rock
Yeah, Yeah.	side to side.
Can you go "sh-sh?"	Whisper "sh-sh."
Yeah, Yeah.	
Can you go "sh-sh?"	
Yeah, Yeah.	

9–12 months

The nine to twelve month old begins to stand without support, walk with or without support, climbs up and down stairs, and can easily go from standing to sitting. She is able to pick up and handle even small objects. Once again, all most of these babies need is the space and opportunity to use their muscles and develop physical skills, coordination, and agility. However, we still have the group of overfed, overweight, placid, sedentary babies who are not as interested in physical exercise. If your infant fits into this category, every effort must be made to slow down her weight gain and increase her physical activity.

Another factor that helps create a placid, inactive baby (who may or may not be overweight) is overprotection and overconcern with her physical well-being. If you continually discourage physical activity because you are afraid of an accident, you will inadvertently damage and even destroy her natural curiosity—so important for healthy development. Of course, it is necessary to "child-proof" your house. Most accidents can be prevented by removing all the objects that might be dangerous.

It is always a good idea to take her outdoors as often as possible. Many nine to twelve month olds walk with little or no support and such activity should be encouraged. Less carrying around, fewer trips in the carriage together with more walking will help her become more active and agile.

Let me remind you again that babies are sturdy and strong and love roughhouse activities. Wrestling and tumbling develop and strengthen many muscles.

Various sized balls, large enough not to be swallowed or choked on are a fine source of exercise. Footballs are a favorite because they bounce around in every direction. Besides chasing the ball, your baby will start to learn to throw and sometimes even catch it.

An excited father called me during my morning advice hour to report, "You won't believe this, but Joey, who is just 11 months old, caught a rubber ball I threw him three times in a row." I don't know if Joey will play for the New York Yankees someday, but I do know that he's a very well-coordinated little baby, already on the right road toward real fitness. Here are more **Gymboree®** activities for nine-to-twelve-month-olds:

ROW, ROW, ROW YOUR BOAT
(Tune: "Row, Row, Row Your Boat")

Position: Parent on back with knees up. Baby lies on parent's knees, looking down.

Words

Row, row, row your boat
Gently down the stream.
Merrily, merrily,
Merrily, merrily,
Life is but a dream.

2. Rock, rock, rock,
   your boat . . .

Movements

Parent raises and lowers
her legs, lifting the baby
up and down.

Rock baby side to side.

DOVER
(Chant)

Position: Baby lying on back facing parent.

Words

Leg over, leg over,
The dog went to Dover.
When he came to a fence,
Jump! He went over!

Movements

Cross one ankle over other.
Alternate.
Alternate again.
At "jump" lift both legs.

MOVING
(Tune: "Wheels on the Bus")

Position: Baby is lying on back facing parent.

Words

Move your arms up and down
Up and down, up and down.
Move your arms up and down
Here at Gymboree.

2. Touch your fingers and
   your toes . . .

Movements

Raise and lower baby's arms.

Touch fingers together.
Touch toes.

3. Touch your toe
   to your ear . . .   Touch toe to ear.

4. Sit up and then   Sit baby up,
   lay down . . .   lay baby back down.

5. Roll to the left and   Roll baby to left.
   then to the right . . .   Roll baby to right.

SPACE MOUNTAIN

Place four or five inner tubes or GymTubes™ on the floor under a mat. The children can then crawl, walk, or climb over the mat.

CHAPTER 15
Toddler Activities

Though some are more placid than others, all normal toddlers have an intense desire to move around and explore. This built-in drive helps them gain mastery over their bodies, and at the same time allows them to learn more about their environment. Most toddlers, left to their own devices, are absolute dynamos, as any parent will readily attest. "I can't keep up with him," is a common remark made by mothers and fathers of youngsters this age. It is usually said half in admiration and half in complaint.

Of course, a parent can't leave the toddler on his own. He has to be protected from the hot stove and electric wiring, and prevented from tumbling down a flight of stairs. That is just indoors. Outdoors there is a different set of threats to his physical well-being. How many times a day do you say to your toddler, "don't touch" "stay here," watch out," "be careful," "sit still"? You do it because you must. You would be negligent if you did not do your best to keep your child out of harm's way.

Unfortunately, if you are *too* safety conscious, your toddler may begin to get the idea that being still is better than being active. This won't happen right away because his drive to explore is quite strong. It will never happen if you provide a variety of good, safe opportunities for exercise. Your job is to encourage him by offering the opportunities that will motivate him to learn to use his body and ultimately to find the joy in movement that will last into adulthood. But, without those opportunities, plus lots of encouragement from you, your little one may eventually take your admonishments to heart and spend more and more time just sitting around, staying out of trouble.

Television, the great pacifier, now also comes into the picture. At about this age, the child begins to take a greater interest in the programs on the screen, especially if his parents and older siblings are in the habit of spending long hours sitting in front of the TV set. Sometimes it is a great relief to parents when their toddler starts watching television. "Finally," said one young mother, "I can get a little work done without having to worry about what Suzy's up to." It is easy to sympathize with this mother and others like her. Running after a toddler all day long is one of the hardest jobs known to mankind or womankind. Even the most devoted parents sometimes are desperate for a break and, in effect, that is what putting a child in front of a TV set gives them.

I don't think TV is terrible for small children. In this day and age it is a part of everyone's life and so why should it be any different for the toddler? However, it is a very bad idea to allow a young child to spend hours on end in front of the set. Too many hours of TV watching are hours that are better spent in active play.

The toddler who is encouraged to sit quietly for most of each day and whose parents do not allow him to participate in safe, active play is very likely to become a sedentary school-ager who in turn becomes the flabby, out-of-shape adolescent, and who, as an adult will be at greater risk for a host of the ailments that plague our society.

All children need exercise for good health and development, but it is again worthwhile to mention here relationship between exercise and overweight. Many fat toddlers actually eat less than their thinner playmates. This runs counter to conventional wisdom. Everything else being equal, we would expect the child who eats less to weigh less. In this case, everything else is *not* equal. Fat children tend to be less active than thin or normal-weight children. Physical activity burns calories. The more active the child, the greater the number of calories burned over the course of the day. The fat child who consumes 1,200 calories but sits around most of the time might burn off only 1,100 in a 24-hour period. He then ends up with a net gain of 100 calories, which is stored in his body as fat. On the other hand, the thin child who eats 1,400 calories might skip and jump his way through the whole 1,400 calories and more. There is no gain at the end of the day, no fat stored away in his body.

Does obesity lead to the lack of exercise in the toddler? Sometimes. And when it does, it starts a vicious cycle. We know that fat children don't move around as easily as thin ones. They tend to be clumsier and fall down more often. Many fat toddlers already lack stamina. In short, it is more difficult for a child who carries around excess weight to run and jump and play with total abandon.

If your toddler is already overweight, it will not be enough to modify his diet by cutting down on calories. You must also do everything possible to help him increase his physical activity.

I have advised you not to force your toddler or urge him to eat when he doesn't feel hungry, and not to make a fuss if he does not eat the foods you think he ought to have. From long experience, I know that this hands-off policy is best in the long run.

As far as exercise is concerned, however, I don't believe in this hands-off policy. Despite the current adult fitness craze the general trend of our society has been toward greater passivity and a more sedentary lifestyle. Where their own children are concerned, parents must take an active role in reversing these tendencies.

Instead of curbing all your child's impulses to run and jump and tumble and hop, channel them. You can do this by seeing that he has space to play in and a few simple toys. You don't need huge spaces. Small children can play happily in a small house or apartment and, if there is no backyard, they should be taken for regular outings at a playground. You might also want to look into the new franchised children's exercise programs that feature activities planned especially for toddlers. They are listed in the Yellow Pages under "Health Clubs."

The following are some specific suggestions for helping your toddler develop coordination, strength, and agility:

1. *Push and pull toys*: Cars and trucks, often with noises and sound effects built in, make this activity great fun. These toys are useful for both small and large muscle development, and allow the toddler the opportunity to move around and exercise in his make-believe world.

2. *Balls*: Let your toddler play with balls of various sizes. He can learn to throw a ball and even catch it if it is large enough, and he certainly can have a great time kicking the ball around. Balls help hand-eye coordination, agility, and overall coordination.

3. *Crawling games*: These are excellent for large muscle development. Anything you can do to figure out ways to make it fun is splendid exercise. For example, cut out the sides of a large cardboard box such as the one that a television set came in and, lo and behold, he has an indoor and outdoor playhouse!

4. *Roughhouse activities*: Gentle roughhousing is great for parent and toddler. It does not require special equipment except maybe a blanket or pad on the floor. There are no rules. You can do it any time and it uses all the muscles and burns off extra calories. Roughhousing is good for both the child's physical and emotional well-being. Because it is important for you to participate when giving him your full and undivided attention, I suggest that you stop frequently during your wrestling matches for rest periods and big hugs.

5. *Hop and skip games*: This is another splendid parent-child activity. You can do it both indoors or out, although outside your toddler will have a greater opportunity to stretch his legs and really run. Needless to say, you will be ready to quit long before he will.

6. *Outdoor play yard*: If you have your own or a neighbor's yard available, this is ideal. A playground with proper equipment is just as good. Get your toddler outside as often as possible, even when it is cold. There's an old wives' tale that cold air is unhealthy for little children and can cause pneumonia. This is absolutely untrue. If you remember this you will be encouraged to take your toddler outside every chance you get, including the winter. It is unfair to keep an active toddler indoors during the

cold months of the year. The more opportunities he is given to run, jump, and climb, the stronger and healthier he'll be.

7. *Climbers and slides*: These are excellent sources of good exercise and teach your toddler agility and coordination.

8. *Four-wheeled vehicle*: Your toddler can sit on and straddle the vehicle and maneuver himself around. This is fine exercise and helps prepare him for the first tricycle.

9. *Chores*: Toddlers are quite strong and willing and able to work, and so it is good practice to get your child involved in helping around the house. This will improve his physical development as well as help to develop a sense of cooperation. Taking out garbage, moving a small piece of furniture, carrying packages are all chores that are well within his physical capabilities.

10. Also try these songs and games from **Gymboree®** with your toddler.

Toddler Games from **Gymboree®**

HEAD AND SHOULDERS
(Tune: "London Bridge")

Words	*Movements*
Head and shoulders knees and toes, Knees and toes, knees and toes. Head and shoulders knees and toes, Clap your hands and around we go.	Touch head, shoulders, etc. with hands.

STRETCH, STRETCH
(Tune: "Twinkle Twinkle Little Star")

Words	*Movements*
Stretch, stretch away up high On your tiptoes, reach the sky. Put your hands upon your waist Hold them there and make a face. Now bend down and touch your toes Stay right there and touch your nose.	Follow actions indicated by words.

BICYCLE SONG
(Tune: Farmer in the Dell)

Words

We're riding up the hill.
We're riding up the hill.
We're riding slowly up the hill
And then we're riding down.
We're riding down the hill.
We're riding down the hill.
We're riding quickly down the hill
And then we're riding up.

Movements

Children do bicycling movements in either a seated position or up on their shoulders. The first verse is done slowly.
The second verse is done quickly.

RIGHT HAND, LEFT HAND

Words

This is my right hand.
I'll raise it up high.

This is my left hand.
I'll touch the sky.

Right hand,
Left hand,
Roll them around.

Left hand,
Right hand,
Pound, pound, pound.

Movements

Right hand extended.
Raise hand over head.

Left hand extended.
Raise hand over head.

Show right palm.
Show left palm.
Roll forearms.

Show left palm.
Show right palm.
Pound with fists.

Between two and three years of age, toddlers start to enjoy rhythmic play, dancing, and can ride a tricycle. They try very hard to exercise their muscles by involving themselves in all sorts of vigorous activities, such as pulling wagons and toy wheelbarrows. This is an ideal age to start to encourage development of skills in various sports, especially those that he can continue all his life. It still is too early to think about skiing, skating, tennis, or golf, but how about swimming, running, soccer, and wrestling? Swimming is an ideal sport and exercise, and toddlers have no fear of the water. It is important that they not be rushed and that the instruction be supervised by an expert. There are many organized programs available designed especially to teach young children how to swim. Soccer is an excellent sport for the two to three year old, because he can kick a ball and run all day long. At this age your child can probably learn to throw and catch a ball. Throwing and catching with your toddler will improve his hand-eye coordination and get him ready for a number of sports later on, including baseball and basketball. Finally, wrestling is a splendid sport for the two to three year old. It is marvelous fun and an excellent overall conditioner. It helps build up strength, agility, balance, and stamina. All these sports and exercises are appropriate for both boys and girls.

CHAPTER 16
Exercise for Your Preschooler

Once upon a time, not so very many years ago, hardly anyone thought about exercise as a major factor in children's health. There was little need for such concern. Back then, in the days before television, and when crime in the streets and automobile traffic was less of a threat to small children, kids as young as four or five spent the hours from morning until night outdoors with their friends, running, skipping, jumping, rolling in the grass and, in general, using their small bodies to the fullest.

I don't need to tell you how times have changed. Most parents are now reluctant to allow their preschoolers out of doors without close and constant adult supervision. Given the realities of modern life, that is as it should be.

Many mothers are not available to provide that supervision for many hours each day, because they're away at work. These youngsters spend most of their time indoors with a baby-sitter or TV set or at a day-care center or nursery school, in circumstances where there are fewer opportunities for vigorous physical activity. The results are unfortunate. Our children are getting weaker and they're getting fatter and they're developing the sedentary habits which make it more likely that they will develop high blood pressure or become victims of a heart attack or stroke as adults. The irony of it all is that although children

Exercise for Your Preschooler   185

are becoming less and less physically fit, many of the adults in our population are joining health clubs, taking aerobic dance classes, buying rowing machines and stationary bicycles, jogging, and investing great amounts of time and energy in an effort to shape up. As we already have pointed out, the hazards of a sedentary lifestyle are well documented.

It is important for parents to realize that helping their children develop sound exercise habits is at least as important as any other single effort in enhancing present health and insuring long and vigorous futures. The word *effort* is the key one in the preceding sentence: By the time a child is four or five, the bad habits may have already taken hold.

Some preschoolers are already television junkies, and it is not easy to tear them away from the TV set on a Saturday morning for a run in the park. Some, encouraged by loving, well-meaning parents to "sit still and be good" when they were toddlers, already have negative feelings about physical activity. They have learned to be overly quiet and overly cautious where their bodies are concerned.

These "old" habits (if it can be said that the habits of a four or five year old are "old") are not going to be easy to break. Instilling new, healthier exercise habits will require active involvement—*effort*—on the part of the parents. It is difficult to talk a youngster into spending less time in front of the television set on a beautiful Sunday afternoon if you also prefer to spend Sundays in front of the tube. It's almost impossible to convince a lazy five year old that running or playing ball or swimming is fun if you yourself shun these activities.

Parental example is a mighty potent force during these years. Later on, other people, including peers and teachers, will have more influence on your child. Still later, your child will reach a stage in which there is a natural tendency to rebel. When that time comes, your words and actions will count for much less, but for now you are the most important role models. Therefore use your influence to shape her habits in positive ways by becoming more active yourself. If you do, I can almost guarantee that your preschooler will learn to enjoy exercise. Not only that, but *you* too will reap the benefits!

EXERCISE THAT'S FUN AND EASY

Plenty of exercise is a must for all children, but it is particularly beneficial for the fat child. Indeed, the lack of exercise may be the primary reason for her overweight state. Many fat children take in fewer calories per day than their slimmer friends but because the fat child tends to be less active, she burns fewer calories, which are stored as fat. For these children it is not enough to just reduce food intake. They must be encouraged to increase their level of physical activity as well. Only then will the problem of the too-rapid gain be brought under control.

A child of four or five does not need acres of wide open spaces in order to play. If you have no yard of your own, she should be taken regularly to a safe park or playground. If you can find one that has climbing and crawling-through equipment as well as slide and swings, so much the better! The following are some specific suggestions to help your preschooler develop strength, agility, coordination, and stamina.

1. *Swimming*: This is an excellent age to encourage swimming and it certainly is not too early for lessons. Check with your local Y or health club to see when beginner classes are given. With proper instruction, your child will be able to master basic swimming skills and learn proper swimming techniques and water safety. Freestyle water play with you is an excellent activity for preschoolers.

2. *Dance classes*: Lessons in modern jazz, tap, or ballet are popular at this age and provide great opportunities for exercise. Some dance studios also offer basic gymnastics and aerobic classes tailored to the abilities of the preschooler.

3. *Family outings*: Hiking, easy "mountain" climbing (actually hill climbing), and jogging are fun for everyone in the family and well within the capabilities of most preschoolers.

4. *Roughhousing*: Gentle wrestling with a parent is excellent exercise for a four or five year old. It can be done on a bed, on a floor with rug or mat, any time you have a few extra minutes. I am very much in favor of this form of activity, because it exercises all her muscles and increases strength and flexibility, and also because it brings parent and child together in a unique way that is enjoyable for both. Naturally, easy does it on your

part, and don't forget to call for frequent time-outs to rest (if not for your child, surely for you).

5. *Peer games*: It's important to make every effort to have your preschooler spend playtime with friends her own age. If some of this time can be spent outdoors in a safe environment under supervision, plenty of strenuous exercise will naturally follow. Preschoolers are imaginative and invent all sorts of games requiring running, jumping, chasing, tagging, and such. If these exercises get out of hand, organize a miniature soccer game with the group. Soccer is one of the exercises I particularly encourage for children of all ages. It is fast paced and an action sport. It features running, twisting, and jumping, and is ideal to develop true physical fitness together with a nice set of bumps and bruises.

6. *Doing things the hard way*: Anything that gets your preschooler moving and using her muscles counts as exercise. That includes walking with her (instead of driving) to nursery school, the park, or the library. It also includes chores (such as sweeping the floor, making her bed, and taking out the garbage).

7. Try these **Gymboree®** exercises with your preschooler.

ROW YOUR BOAT
(Tune: "Row, Row, Row Your Boat")

Words	*Movements*
Row Row Row your boat Gently down the stream. Ha ha I fooled you I'm a submarine!	Parent and child sit facing each other and hold hands. Rock back and forth. Let go of hands and both lie back.

OPEN, SHUT THEM
(Tune: "Open, Shut Them")

Words	Movements
Open, shut them, Open shut them. Make a little clap, clap, clap.	Children open and shut hands held high over their heads.
Open, shut them, Open, shut them. Give a little stamp, stamp, stamp.	Jump legs apart, together. Repeat. Stamp feet.
Creep them, creep them Slowly creep them. Like a little mouse.	Tiptoe to the center of circle.
Stretch them, stretch them, Great big stretch them. Run around the house!	Take big steps back to original position. Take quick steps around the circle.

The goal of the Eden Fitness Program is to raise a healthier, stronger, more vigorous child who will grow up with fewer risk factors for the deadly, degenerative diseases of adult life. If you take the steps to insure that your preschool-age child follows the exercise guidelines we have discussed in this chapter, she will already be well on her way to achieving maximum physical fitness.

CHAPTER 17
Exercise and Sports for Your School-Ager

On the very morning I sat down to write this section, I heard on the radio that a group of Harvard researchers reported that the incidence of obesity was higher among kids who spent greater than usual amounts of time watching television. Well, thank you, researchers, for confirming what most of us knew all along—or should have. The body that sits for long hours on end in front of the TV set burns up fewer calories than an active body. Extra calories that are not burned up are converted into fat, which is stored away in fat cells. If enough fat is stored away into these cells, the result is obesity. It's as simple as that.

The link between inactivity and obesity is very clear. Lack of exercise is as much a cause of overweight as overeating. Certainly, the surest way to "cure" fat is to start a program combining a lower-calorie diet with an increase in physical activity.

The fat child must become more active if he is ever to slim down. Normal-weight kids who are sedentary must also step up their level of physical activity if they are to grow up strong and healthy. As I discussed in the chapter on exercise, lack of exercise (whether a person is fat or not) is an important risk factor in the development of high blood pressure, stroke, and heart attack. Of course, your child is not likely to be a victim of any of these medical disasters in his school years, but if he is sedentary now and remains so as an adult, his chances of becoming a victim go way up.

Unfortunately, although we are in the midst of a fitness boom among adults, among the kids there seems to be a fitness bust. Quoting from Dr. Paul Dyment, Chairman of the Sports Medicine Committee of the American Academy of Pediatrics, "One of the great ironies of American life is that many parents are now frequently more fit than their child."

A recent U.S. Department of Health and Human Services study of 8,800 children indicates that youngsters today tend to be slightly fatter than their parents were in the 1960s and that only about 50 percent of American school-aged children get enough exercise to develop healthy hearts and lungs. In San Francisco, more than a third of a group of youngsters from low-income families studied were unable to complete even 10 minutes of moderate exercise without becoming exhausted, whereas in Florida, students given fitness tests did not score as well as the children given the same fitness test nine years earlier. Our children are running to fat and flab, and it seems to be getting worse.

I have said it elsewhere in this book but it's worth repeating here: Getting your child to be more active is one of the most important things you can do to protect his health and enhance his physical well-being. Your child will never become truly fit without a regular sensible exercise plan.

"Between her piano lessons, French lessons, and homework, Amy is just too busy to get any exercise," the mother of a nine year old recently told me. This was in response to my explaining to her just how important it was that Amy become more physically active. Usually when I ask parents to think more carefully about what their children do all day long, they discover that there are some fairly large blocks of free time that could be used for exercise. Amy's mother, on reconsidering her daughter's weekday routine, realized that she did most of her homework with friends and was almost always finished before 5:00 P.M. The hour between 5:00 and 6:00 was often spent on the telephone or watching TV. Dinner was usually over by 6:30 and was followed by more TV until 9:30, Amy's bedtime. On an ordinary day, Amy had plenty of time to exercise, after all. Her mother had overestimated how busy her daughter was, and my guess is that many other parents do the same. I recognize that many youngsters do live with intense time pressures. There are those with paper routes, or other part-time jobs, those who take additional regular after-school instruction, and those who must travel long distances to get back and forth to school. Nevertheless, time must be found for vigorous physical exercise and activity on a regular basis.

It upsets me when parents claim that their school-age children are just too tired for physical activity. Nonsense! Lots of healthy school-agers are too lazy, too set in their sedentary ways, too mesmerized by the "idiot" box to bestir themselves, but too tired? Never!! If a child gets enough sleep and there is nothing physically wrong with him, a half hour of brisk exercise each day won't strain the poor fellow. In fact, it has been shown that moderate exercise, far from causing exhaustion, actually tends to *add* to a person's store of energy.

Time problems rarely explain why a youngster won't exercise. Neither is "tiredness" a factor. Rather, it is lack of motivation that keeps most kids from being active, together with the sedentary habits that have been developing since toddlerhood— habits that have kept them sitting around instead of running, jumping, swimming, skating, and participating in sports that help develop their bodies' fullest potential of fitness.

Your job as parents is to provide motivation to overcome the old sedentary patterns. This is not an easy task. It means that if you yourself are not active, you are going to have to turn over a new leaf and provide a better example for your youngster. School-agers like to be with their friends, but "playing" with mother or dad or both still appeals to them. Let me warn you now, however, that this state of affairs will be over within a few short years when your child becomes a teen-ager. But for now, if you can find just a half hour a day to walk, jog, bicycle, swim, or just dance around the living room with your child, both of you will reap enormous benefits in terms of increased fitness and better health. There are also great emotional advantages to exercising with your child, because sharing in this kind of activity will inevitably draw you closer together. Children always remember the happy times they spend together with their parents.

What if you can't find the time for physical exercise with your school-ager no matter how hard you try? Then you will have to be inventive and devise other ways to get him moving. Arrange skating and swimming parties for him and his friends. Organize a softball, soccer, or basketball game. Anything and everything that requires him to use his muscles counts as exercise, even household chores such as vacuuming, making beds, or walking the dog.

That reminds me of a fat ten year old I once treated without success. His parents were also fat and had a hard time sticking to the changes that had to be made in the family diet. Dan's weight continued to climb with each monthly visit until suddenly there was a 2-pound weight loss over the previous month. I congratulated his mother for finally implementing the diet guidelines I had given her. She answered somewhat sheepishly that they were all still eating the same old way. Puzzled, I insisted that something must have changed in her son's life, otherwise how could we account for the weight loss? Neither mother nor child could offer an explanation. The next month they arrived at my office with a beautiful, active golden retriever. You guessed it. My young patient was burning off hundreds of extra calories each day running and playing with his new companion.

There is no vitamin or magic exercise pill that will make up for a sedentary lifestyle. There is no way a child can achieve optimal health and fitness without being physically active. Therefore I believe it is entirely appropriate for you to insist that he get up and get moving. Exercise with him, arrange for him to engage in vigorous activity with friends. Give him chores. Do everything you can to provide opportunities for him to use his body and the sooner you get started the better.

SCHOOL-AGE EXERCISE OPTIONS

A child between the ages of six and ten is physically capable of participating in an enormous range of activities. Your job as a parent is to help him explore all the available options. He won't like everything he tries of course, but he doesn't have to. If you can steer him toward just a couple of physical activities he enjoys, you will be doing fine.

It is important to concern yourselves with the physical education programs in your child's school. It might be a good idea to get other parents interested in visiting the school with you to be certain the program provides at least one hour of physical activity and exercise every day plus organized after-school sports. In my experience, there are far too many schools whose physical education programs leave much to be desired.

This is the age for outdoor group games such as tag, dodge ball, and kick-the-can. Rope jumping is an excellent exercise both in terms of burning up calories and in terms of developing agility, coordination, and strength.

This is the time to help your child start learning a "carry-over" sport, a sport that he can continue to play the rest of his life. Good examples of "carry-over" sports are swimming, skating, bowling, biking, and tennis. The two sports I excelled in as a school-ager were tennis and baseball. The last baseball game I ever played was in my senior year at college. I have continued to play tennis all my life, however, and am still at it today. If your child learns the skills of a "carry-over" sport now, he will be proficient enough by the time he is an adolescent to want to continue. If you wait, it won't be easy to push your reluctant teen-ager into action. A few tennis lessons by a professional to learn proper stroke techniques will be well worth the cost. "Carry-over" sports establish lifelong and life-enhancing exercise habits.

Another excellent sport that both boys and girls can participate in is soccer; it is relatively safe and the size and weight of the child is not important. My best advice is to expose your child to as many sports as possible so that he may find the one or two that he will continue to participate in as he grows up. Early morning workout shows (or exercise video cassettes) in which the instructor leads the viewer through calisthenics and aerobic maneuvers in the privacy of the home may be just the thing for the child who is reluctant to exercise in public. For this reason, I highly recommend video workouts for the very fat and/or awkward school-ager who might otherwise get no exercise at all.

Dance classes from jazz to tap, to modern, to ballet, are terrific exercises and often are very appealing to shyer children who feel uncomfortable with the noisy competitiveness of team sports. The same is true of gymnastics and acrobatic classes.

School-age children are ready to learn and participate in a wide variety of competitive sports, such as softball, touch football, basketball, soccer, ice hockey, volleyball, and so a few words of caution may be in order: If your child is awkward or has not already attained some competence in a sport, don't force him into competition with children who are more advanced. Rather, see if you can round up and organize a group of youngsters whose skills are on a par with his. Keep in mind that practice in these sports is just as valuable or may be more valuable in getting your child to exercise than playing an actual game. If your child enjoys softball, for example, he will no doubt get more exercise from a half hour of pitching or fielding practice with you than during a full seven innings of team play.

Family outings are another exercise option that you should consider. I have found that children who do best at exercise usually come from families that pursue physical activity as a group. When everyone sets off to swim, bowl, ski, or jog, when the whole family hikes through the woods or skis together, they not only enjoy each other's company, but they also burn off calories and strengthen muscles. Of course, most families can't engage in any of these activities often enough to obtain maximum fitness benefits. Never mind that. Even the occasional day or weekend spent out of doors in constant motion with your school-ager can be an excellent exercise bonus.

Finally, an important exercise option is household chores. I have already mentioned vacuuming and bed making as good way to get your school-agers moving and using their muscles. But they're not the only chores that are valuable in this regard. Others are washing floors and windows, mopping or sweeping with a broom, folding laundry, putting away dishes and groceries, and scrubbing pots and pans. Need I point out that another advantage of chores as exercise is less work for mom and dad.

An essential ingredient of the Eden Fitness Program is exercise. No matter how nutritious a diet you supply your child, without sufficient exercise he will not achieve maximum physical fitness. Without proper exercise, he will become much more vulnerable to many serious illnesses. If your school-aged child has always been active, be grateful and see to it that he continues to remain physically active. If your school-ager has basically led a sedentary life up until now, you had better get busy. Your job is to get him up off his derriere and help him start developing proper exercise habits that he will continue as he grows into adolescence and beyond.

CHAPTER 18
Exercise and Sports for Your Adolescent

The teen years have traditionally been a time of never-ending activity, including gym class at school, competitive after-school sports, bicycling, swimming, skating, dancing, outdoor outings of various kinds, and perhaps a part-time job requiring physical labor.

That is the way it was when I was young and perhaps it was that way for you, as well. Apparently, however, physical activity plays a less important role in the lives of vast members of today's adolescents.

According to the number of recent studies, including the three-year U.S. Department of Health and Human Services Survey of children in grades five through twelve teen-agers in the 1980s are less active and thus not as strong and fit as their counterparts of a decade ago. Lack of exercise also helps explain the fact that today's teen-agers tend to be somewhat fatter than two decades ago.

If the only benefit of physical activity was to develop strong, toned-up muscles, it might be easier to overlook all the data suggesting that American teen-agers are under-exercised. Exercise does far more than simply build up muscles, however. In fact, as more and more research is carried out it becomes clearer that sufficient exercise is just as important as proper diet in achieving optimal fitness and health.

Take the case of exercise as it relates to overweight. Many fat youngsters eat less than children of normal weight. Because normal-weight kids are more active and burn off the calories they take in, however, they don't accumulate unhealthy pounds of fat. Overweight teen-agers, on the other hand, are often "sitters." They don't move around very much and thus don't get rid of many of the calories they consume. The excess is stored as fat. Obese teen-agers *must* realize that if they are to slim down, they must not only begin to eat differently but they must also exercise more. Diet without exercise never works, especially for the overweight adolescent.

The benefits of exercise go way beyond the prevention and treatment of obesity. A half hour of vigorous physical activity three to four times a week over a period of eight months, for example, has been shown to lower blood pressure in preteens and teen-agers significantly, according to a recent report in *Pediatric News*. Because blood pressure tends to rise with advancing age, lower blood pressure early in life reduces the risk of hypertension later on, and thus helps protect against future heart attacks and strokes.

The role of exercise in increasing heart and lung health is well known. The result—cardiovascular fitness—is what all of us should strive for. It also raises the "fatigue threshold," making it possible to accomplish more while feeling less tired. In other words, it increases stamina and strength. As far as the two components of the Eden Fitness Program—*nutrition* and *exercise*—the teen-ager probably will benefit more from the exercise.

Less familiar to many is the effect of regular exercise on psychological health and well-being. Researchers have noted a remarkable improvement in attitude, self-image, and self-esteem in teen-agers who exercise regularly, reports Dr. Bert M. Franks, of the Texas Christian University Health Center, Fort Worth, Texas. I have been well aware of the emotional and psychological benefits of exercise in all my adolescent patients, not just in the fat ones.

It is hard to think of a bigger health "bargain" for an adolescent (or anyone else for that matter) than exercise. It can make you look better, work better, feel better (and, according to some studies, even think better), whereas at the same time it helps prevent some serious medical problems. Not only that, it is free! Of course, if an activity requires special equipment or professional lessons, the cost can be considerable. But brisk walking and jogging, two excellent forms of exercise that everybody can do, come absolutely free of charge. Another point to remember is that achieving fitness through proper exercise does not take a great deal of time. Thirty minutes, three or four times a week does it.

I have met few parents of adolescents who, after hearing me describe the benefits of exercise, did not completely agree with me. If all I had to do was to convince the parents of my patients of the importance of regular exercise, all their teen-agers would be fit as a fiddle—but it's not that easy.

Exercise is just like diet. By the time a youngster reaches the age of eleven or twelve it is no longer possible to oversee and direct all or most of her activities. It becomes very difficult to *make* your child get up earlier in the morning to run for half an hour. You can't force her to do sit-ups at bedtime. You can't force her to do the Jane Fonda workout.

All you can do is *encourage* her to be more active. One of the best ways is to embark on a fitness program of your own. This may work despite the fact that adolescence is considered a time of rebellion against the values of the older generation. Many teen-agers I have taken care of become more interested in exercise after they have seen their own parents take it up. Why? It may be associated with the competitiveness of wanting to outdo mother or father. If dad can jog a mile in good time, junior wants to prove that he can do it also—but faster!

Another way to encourage your adolescent to step up her physical activity is to remove the obstacles in her path, make it easier for her, in other words. If she enjoys swimming, get her a membership at a regular Y and find out which hours, if any, are reserved for teen-agers. If her bike is broken, get it fixed. If she has outgrown her old ice skates, buy her a new pair (just say it's an early birthday or Christmas present). If she's fat and embarrassed about it, don't push her into joining activities with normal-weight children her own age. Rather, suggest but don't insist that she exercise on her own. Ask her to tune in to one of the early-morning TV workout shows so she can exercise in the privacy of her own home.

As we have discussed in earlier chapters, household chores can be good exercise. Assign her a variety of lawn, yard, or household tasks, including washing or waxing the car, raking or mowing, painting a room, waxing floors, and so on; all require physical exertion and entail a good expenditure of energy.

If you have been driving her everywhere up to now, stop. She's old enough to walk and the additional use of her muscles will be good for her. I remember giving this advice to the mother of a lazy seventeen-year-old teen-ager who was not fat but was far from fit. "I don't drive her anywhere, Dr. Eden, she has her own car."

Suggest that she get a part-time job. Obviously work, with kids her age, moving and using her body, is desirable in terms of providing exercise benefits. But *any* job that takes her out of the house and keeps her up is preferable to having her lounge around at home watching endless hours of TV. Nowadays, besides TV, we have home computers and video games, two more factors that contribute to the S.O.B. syndrome that we discussed in Chapter 7.

Some teen-agers need just a bit of encouragement to become more active. Once they take the initial steps they soon discover that using their bodies can be fun. In time, exercise becomes a habit, perhaps the healthiest, most life-enhancing habit of all. Others react far more negatively, often the fat ones. They moan, they groan, they resist with all their might. The teen-agers who are most averse to exercise are precisely the ones who need it most. If your child falls into this category, especially if she has always been sedentary, you will have a hard time trying to change her ways. Screaming and yelling won't do it. Set the proper example yourself and gently encourage her to join in. Perhaps suggest that she read the chapter on exercise.

The aerobic exercises listed here are most beneficial in terms of achieving true physical fitness. They don't require partners or teams:

1. Brisk walking
2. Jogging
3. Running
4. Cycling
5. Rope jumping
6. Lap swimming
7. Aerobic dancing

As we have pointed out, these aerobic exercises are the ones that promote true cardiovascular fitness. If done on a regular basis, meaning for 30 minutes at least three times per week, your teen-ager will be well on her way to true physical fitness.

If your child, during her school-age years developed skills in one or two "carry-over" sports, now is the time to encourage her to continue. We're referring to sports such as swimming, skating, biking, and tennis. If she hasn't done much up to now, there is still plenty of time to learn. If your fourteen-year-old daughter has never picked up a tennis racket up to now, it's unlikely that she'll ever become another Chris Evert Lloyd, but so what? With a series of lessons from a competent tennis pro she can still learn the game. Then, if she practices enough, she'll be able to play a good game and enjoy it, now, during her teen years, and for the rest of her life. Some of these late bloomers do very well. One of our group didn't take up tennis until he was forty, and he's very tough for me to beat even though I've been playing all my life.

Competitive school sports are an important part of many teen-agers' lives. If that is the case with your child, I think it's great. The more the merrier, as long as there is proper supervision and equipment, and as long as your child has the physical capabilities appropriate to the sport. I remember discussing the advisability of football for a large, overweight, late-maturing fourteen-year-old boy whose father was very anxious that he try out for the team. He thought that because John was big and heavy he would be a perfect candidate for a defensive lineman. I explained that John wasn't ready. Because of John's late skeletal maturity and muscle mass, he didn't yet have the strength or endurance and so would perform poorly and be at greater risk of a significant injury if he played competitive football too soon. I recommended that this large, obese, late maturer avoid collision sports and rather get started on a weight control and fitness program. After trimming down and becoming fit and suitably mature, perhaps in a year or two he would be ready to become a candidate for football.

Exercise, like diet, is far too important to be left to chance or to your teen-agers' personal preferences. The Eden Fitness Program does not suggest that you try to turn her into a super-athlete or perfect physical specimen. What we do suggest is that you help her manage to effect a modest increase in physical activity.

Your teen-ager will soon be an adult, out on her own. These adolescent years are difficult ones, both for the teen-ager and for her parents. It is easy to throw up your hands and abdicate your role during these turbulent, emotional years. It is more difficult to stand fast and try to help develop healthy exercise habits in your adolescent. Obviously, it is much easier if a fitness program is started when your child is very young. Changing a sedentary lifestyle that has developed over many years takes some doing. If you find yourself in this situation, don't be discouraged. You won't make progress very rapidly, but then again, Rome wasn't built in a day. Little by little inroads will be made. By sticking with it, you will have an excellent chance of helping your teen-ager achieve physical fitness. By making even modest modifications in her exercise patterns you will be giving her a tremendous advantage in terms of her future well-being and health. You will lower the risk of future heart attack, stroke, high blood pressure, and nutrition-related cancers. This is the best present you can ever give your teenager.

PART IV
NUTRITION FOR THE OVERWEIGHT CHILD

CHAPTER 19
Why It's Important to Be Slim

About the same percentage of children and adults are fat: about 30 percent of all children and 30 percent of all adults. The $64,000 question is whether or not it is the same 30 percent. In other words, do fat children grow up to be the fat adults? Of course, the answer is that all of them do not, but most of them do. More often than not, the markedly overweight child grows up to become the fat adult.

Why is it important to raise a normal-weight or thin child? Why is it important to slim down an already overweight schoolager or adolescent? The dangers of adult obesity are well known. The fat adult is at higher risk to develop a stroke or heart attack, and is also at greater risk for certain forms of cancer. But the dangers of childhood obesity are not as well known and so many parents don't worry enough about it. Childhood obesity is unhealty for many reasons. There is a definite association between childhood obesity and elevated blood cholesterol levels. Long-term studies have shown that weight gain in children is the most clear-cut and consistent factor in predicting high blood pressure. Most children found to have hypertension are obese. There is evidence from many sources that fat children are discriminated against in schools, sometimes as early as in kindergarten.

The longer a child is fat the more likely that child will always remain fat. And so the most serious danger of childhood obesity is that it increases the chances of that person being fat as an adult, with all its obvious negative health consequences. The recidivism or relapse rate in the treatment of adult obesity is over 95 percent. This means that less than 5 out of every 100 fat adults are able to maintain their weight loss. Over 95 out of every 100 obese adults gained back all the weight they lost when reexamined two to five years later.

What are the causes of obesity? The basic equation that always holds true is that if you take in more calories than you burn up, the extra calories end up as fat. Every extra 3,500 calories equals one pound of fat. This means that if each day you consume 500 more calories than you burn up, you will gain one pound after seven days ($500 \times 7 = 3,500$). This basic equation does not explain why some children get fat much more easily than others, however, nor does it explain why it is so much more difficult for some children to lose weight than others.

There are four main factors leading to childhood obesity. These are: genetic, metabolic, exercise, and eating patterns.

GENETIC FACTORS

Fat runs in families. Studies have shown that a child born of two obese parents has an 80 percent chance of also being fat. If only one parent is fat, there is a 50 percent chance of that child ending up obese. Children born to two thin parents only have a 10 percent chance of becoming fat. Research on identical twins raised in different environments and studies of adopted children furnish the strongest evidence proving the genetic component of obesity. The identical twin studies showed that as adults each set of twins ended up close in weight as adults even though they were raised separately. The studies of adopted children demonstrated that if two fat people adopt a child born of two thin natural parents, that child's chances of becoming fat are much lower than if she was the natural child of two fat parents. In the book, *Twins: A Study of Heredity and Environment*, the research of H. H. Newman and his colleagues dealt with a comparison of the average differences of body weight of identical twins versus fraternal twins. Their data showed that as adults, only 2 percent of identical twins differed by more than 12 pounds as compared with over 50 percent of the fraternal twins.

The true reason for the genetic factor of obesity is as yet unclear. One theory is that the appetite-regulating center found in the part of the brain called the hypothalamus, may be genetically set. Doctor Norman Jolife, a pioneer in nutrition and obesity, named this center the "appestat." Perhaps the "appestat" is preset so that some families may have genetically determined larger appetites. Another theory is that some newborns are inherently or genetically susceptible to excess production of insulin and HGH (human growth hormone) which, triggered by overnutrition, may encourage excess fat storage in the body.

Another important genetic factor is body build. We all know that body build or body type often runs in families. A small group of the general population are *ectomorphs*—people who have relatively small bodies with long arms and legs and with long, tapered fingers. Ectomorphs usually have small appetites and no matter how much they eat they are unlikely to become fat. On the other hand, *endomorphs* tend to be shorter, softer, and rounder, with short extremities, and they often have great difficulty in maintaining normal weight. Endomorphs deposit fat very easily and so must work much harder to prevent becoming fat. Aside from the total body build configuration, the proportion of some parts of the body also may run in families. For example, some families have a tendency toward large buttocks, thick legs, or heavy breasts—all making it more difficult to maintain body weight.

In terms of preventing obesity, nothing can be done about the genetic factor. After all, your child didn't have the luxury of choosing his parents. But if your family is predisposed to obesity, you will have to be especially vigilant about following the Eden Fitness Program to limit potential health problems.

METABOLIC FACTORS

There are two metabolic mechanisms that may turn out to be important in explaining why some people become fat more easily than others—brown fat and the sodium-potassium pump. Both of these metabolic mechanisms are involved in how quickly and efficiently calories are burned up. They are both less efficient in people who are fat and sedentary than in people who are thin and active.

Brown Fat:

There are two types of fat in the body, yellow fat and brown fat. The yellow fat is stored inert in fat cells and mobilized for energy when needed. It is located all over the body, but is most evident just beneath the skin. Anyone on a diet is trying to get rid of yellow fat. Brown fat is totally different. The body has only a small supply of brown fat as compared with the vast store of yellow fat. Brown fat is located only between the shoulder blades, under the armpits, and around the large veins and arteries close to the heart. Its main function is to warm the vital internal organs, especially the heart. It warms the cold blood moving toward the heart and so prevents the heart from getting chilled. Cold blood reaching the heart can cause dangerous heart rhythm irregularities.

In order to function efficiently, this tiny amount of brown fat must be able to generate tremendous amounts of heat. The fuel that brown fat uses to manufacture this heat is the yellow fat. The more efficient the brown fat, the more fuel (yellow fat) is burned up. As a rule, the brown fat on thin active people burns up many more calories than does the brown fat of obese inactive people.

The more exercise, the more efficient is brown fat metabolism in burning up extra calories. The rise in body heat that takes place for about 4 to 6 hours after vigorous exercise is probably due to the brown fat response. Although there may be a genetically determined difference in brown fat efficiency from person to person, adequate exercise can rev up anybody's brown fat activity, resulting in the burning up of unneeded extra pounds of fat.

Sodium-Potassium Pump:

This is the second metabolic mechanism that seems to be important in relation to obesity (usually referred to as the sodium pump). It is an extremely complicated mechanism whereby sodium is pumped out of the cell and potassium is drawn into the cell. Sodium and potassium continually pass in and out of cells through cell membranes all over the body, and *energy* is continuously being burned in this pumping process.

Doctor George Blackburn of the Harvard Medical School has done a good deal of research in this area. He believes that the sodium pump system works more efficiently in thin active people than in those who are fat and sedentary. The calorie-burning capacity of the sodium pump is lower in the overweight and inactive and higher in the thin and active. This may help explain why many fat people consume fewer calories than their thin peers and still remain fat. If their sodium pumps are less efficient, they burn up fewer calories and thus find it very difficult to get rid of excess fat. Perhaps sluggish sodium pump systems run in families, we just don't know as yet. *Exercise*, however, has been shown to improve the efficiency of the sodium pump system. This is yet another possible explanation for the success of a diet plus exercise program in treating the obese, and the reason why diet alone often fails.

EXERCISE FACTORS

There are some misconceptions about exercise, which are often used to minimize the important role it plays in preventing and treating obesity. The first is that exercise results in very little caloric expenditure. This one can easily be discounted by the fact that daily caloric requirements vary tremendously from the sedentary person, who requires less than 2,000 calories per day, to the very active person (e.g., a marathon runner) who needs 6,000 calories or more per day. And all of us know that marathon runners are among the leanest people in the population.

Exercise plays a very important role in the balance between energy intake and energy output. Doctor William Crosby of Wayne State University School of Medicine in Detroit, recently published an article in the *Journal of the American Medical Association*. He quoted those exercise critics who claim that a person has to walk for more than 36 hours or chop wood for 7 hours or play volleyball for 12 hours just to lose one pound of fat. Using these extremes of exercise, these critics question the effectiveness of weight loss through exercise. The fallacy of this argument is that the calories lost (3,500) depend entirely on one exercise continued for unreasonably long periods of time. If exercise is to be effective in the treatment of obesity, its effects must be cumulative and stretched over reasonable time spans. For example, if the 7 hours of chopping wood is divided into 20 minutes each day, one pound of fat would be lost in three weeks, and 5 pounds in less than 4 months—not bad at all.

Another common myth is that exercise increases appetite and so all the calories burned up during the exercise period are quickly regained during the next meal. This just is not true. Both rat and human experiments show that moderate to vigorous exercise actually decreases the appetite. Quoting from Dr. Jules Hersch from Rockefeller University, "Exercise has a euphoria effect that cuts down the need to turn to food for emotional satisfaction."

A sedentary child burns up no more than 200 to 300 calories above her resting metabolic rate (RMR). Exercise markedly increases the RMR, not only during the actual period of exercise but, as an added bonus, for several hours after the exercise is over. Despite what many believe, the RMR is not much different between thin and fat people (the old "sluggish-thyroid" excuse for obesity).

The evidence is overwhelming that obesity seldom can be prevented or treated successfully if the child does not exercise on a regular basis. Doctor Jean Mayer, the famous nutrition expert, has stated that "probably no single factor is more frequently responsible for the development of obesity—than lack of physical exercise. . . . Repeated studies have shown that the majority of obese adolescents eat less than the average non-obese adolescent of the same sex. Inactivity is likely the reason for the increased percentage of obese youngsters today." Doctor Mayer and his colleagues studied a group of obese girls and found that on average they ate less than the thin control group, but spent only one-third as much time in physical activity. Movies were taken of thin and fat girls swimming and playing tennis, and these films were most revealing. The fat girls hardly moved around on the tennis court and would swing the racket only if the ball happened to bounce somewhere near them. On the other hand, the thin girls scampered all over the court, stretching and leaping to reach the ball. In the swimming pool the obese girls spent most of the exercise period peacefully floating around, occasionally taking a leisurely stroke or two. The thin girls were continually in motion, swimming laps. When the fat girls were questioned, they honestly believed that they had done a lot of real exercise. The truth of the matter was that they had barely exercised at all.

I came across an interesting quote from Dr. Ruth L. Hunemann of the University of California School of Health. "The problem . . . is not eating too much. Rather, it is eating too much for the energy expended. A generally low level of physical activity that appears to be characteristic of American youth and the consequent low caloric need make increased activity an essential part of the regimens for obesity prevention and control." That is why exercise is such an important part of the Eden Fitness Program. Any weight control program must include exercise. With a combined diet and exercise plan, 98 percent of the weight loss is actually fat tissue, whereas with diet alone, only 75 percent of the weight loss is body fat.

The following table lists a number of recreational exercises and household chores appropriate for children, the caloric expenditure for 30 minutes, and the monthly weight loss resulting from the activity. Keep in mind that it requires burning up 3,500 calories to lose one pound of fat.

CALORIE-BURNING ACTIVITIES

	30 minutes	Weight loss per month (approx.)
Walking briskly	175 cal.	1½ lbs.
Jogging	225 cal.	2 lbs.
Running	450 cal.	3½ lbs.
Swimming	340 cal.	3 lbs.
Roller skating	325 cal.	2⅔ lbs.
Biking	250 cal.	2 lbs.
Tennis	250 cal.	2 lbs.
Lawn mowing	230 cal.	2 lbs.
Sweeping floors	75 cal.	¾ lbs.
Bed making	150 cal.	1⅓ lbs.

These numbers prove that a daily regular period of increased physical activity, whether exercise or chores, is essential to prevent and treat childhood obesity.

EATING PATTERNS

Whether it is the toddler who is bribed and rewarded to eat her vegetables with offers of candies and cookies, or the schoolager who eats huge quantities of junk food snacks between meals, or the adolescent who survives on fast-foods and after-dinner binge eating, the results are always the same. These children are eating more calories than their bodies need, and these extra calories, if not burned off by enough physical activity, deposit and form fat tissue.

It has been estimated that the average child in the United States takes in over 30 percent of her daily total calories from between-meal snack foods, many with little or no nutritive value.

CALORIC VALUES OF POPULAR SNACKS

	Calories
Orange soda (8 oz.)	126
Chocolate Popsicle	106
Candy-coated chocolate candies (1 oz.)	130
Potato chips (1 oz.)	158
Peanut brittle (1 oz.)	125
Coconut cookies (5)	390
Pecan brownies (2 oz.)	224
Chocolate chip cookies (5)	250
Ring Ding (2½ oz.)	366
Fruit drink (8 oz.)	110

If a child becomes accustomed to a diet that is too high in "empty" sugar calories, it will be very difficult to get rid of this craving. These sugar-laden foods taste too good, and the child finds it difficult to stop after just a few bites. Rather, she eats large quantities and so takes in excessive calories. A high-fat diet also contributes to obesity. Because one ounce of fat has more than twice the number of calories of one ounce of carbohydrate or protein, less fat needs to be eaten to put on an equal amount of weight. One ounce of protein or carbohydrate has 120 calories, whereas one ounce of fat has 270 calories. The Eden diet is low in both refined sugar and fat.

Early onset obesity, the kind that develops during childhood, is much more difficult to treat than late onset obesity, the kind that starts in adulthood. We don't know for sure why this is so, but perhaps it is the huge number of fat cells that have multiplied during the fat child's periods of rapid growth (the first two years of life and the adolescent growth spurt). Could it be the sedentary lifestyles that these fat children develop? Maybe because the development of faulty feeding habits early in life is so difficult to change later on? Perhaps some metabolic processes within the body slow down during these years of being fat and inactive and cannot be turned up again as an adult. Whatever the reason or reasons, the fact remains that the longer a child is fat, the greater will be her chance of always being fat.

CHAPTER 20 Meals for Fat Toddlers

If your toddler weighs in at just about normal for her age and height, you might be tempted to skip this discussion of fat and what to do about it. I would advise you not to do so. A nutritional pattern that includes too much of the wrong foods often starts during these early years, and too much of the wrong foods may eventually cause even a relatively thin toddler to become too fat. In the case of obesity as in so many other areas of life, an ounce of prevention is worth a pound of cure (no pun intended).

Research done by Dr. Jerome L. Knittle at Mt. Sinai Medical Center in New York concluded that people who have been fat since childhood have an abnormally high number of fat cells or "adipose" cells stored in their bodies. Further, the earlier in life obesity begins, the greater the number of fat cells manufactured. The unfortunate thing about these cells is that once you have them they never go away—not even if the obese child or adult manages to get down to normal weight. Though the fat cells shrink as their fat content is depleted, they always remain ready to fill up with fat again at the slightest opportunity. It is almost as if these cells *crave* fat and *need* to be filled. Although we don't know exactly why, it has been shown time and time again that children and adults with an abnormally large number of these cells find it very difficult to lose weight and, when they do, they usually gain it back again within a short period of time.

The fat cell count for the thin or normal-weight child remains relatively constant between the ages of two and ten. But the fat child continues to manufacture more and more fat cells at a rapid rate. One of the major conclusions of Dr. Knittle and other researchers is that the first five years of life are critical in terms of fat-cell development. Clearly, if you want your toddler to grow up healthy, you must see to it that she does not manufacture extra fat cells. You do this by keeping her thin. Good nutrition and lots of exercise are the keys to keeping your little one's fat-cell count in the normal range. There is another potential bonus benefit: If excessive numbers of fat cells do not develop during these critical years, and if at the same time healthful food and exercise patterns are established, your child probably will never have to deal with the health risks and emotional problems associated with obesity.

But what if she is already fat—a sure indication that even at the age of one or two or three there are abnormal numbers of fat cells? Nothing can be done about the existing fat cells. But you *can* prevent further fat-cell increase by starting to change her diet and exercise habits.

Some parents of fat toddlers are eager to see rapid, dramatic, and visible results of a weight control problem. I remember outlining the Eden Fitness Program to one particularly svelte young mother who was concerned about her chubby two year old. When I told her that the goal was to keep her daughter from gaining weight as quickly as in the past, she protested, "I want Ruth to *lose* weight." That is not the way it works, at least as far as this pediatrician is concerned. I certainly sympathize with a mother's desire for her toddler to slim down, and I heartily applaud her resolve to help the youngster achieve this. But what needs to be pointed out is that a diet low enough in calories to result in a weight loss is often also too low in the nutrients a toddler requires for healthy development. For this reason the goal for the overweight toddler should not be weight loss but rather weight stabilization. Think of it this way: A two year old of average height is fat if she weighs in at 30 pounds. If, through sensible diet and increased exercise, she gains only 5 pounds the next year, then at the age of three she will weigh 35 pounds—still not normal, but she's getting there. If she gains just another 5 pounds during the following year, she will weigh 40 pounds at age four, which is just about right.

Our hypothetical toddler did not lose an ounce, yet through a program of healthy diet and exercise, which slowed her rate of weight gain, the desired results were achieved. Her nutritional needs were not short-changed and over the years good food and exercise habits were being established—habits that will make it less likely for her to develop certain serious illnesses as an adult and habits that will also protect her from the physical and emotional consequences of childhood obesity.

MEAL PLANS FOR OVERWEIGHT TODDLERS

The following menus were designed for the special needs of overweight toddlers.

MONDAY

BREAKFAST	⅓ cup dry oatmeal cooked in water ½ cup low-fat milk ½ tsp. molasses ½ cup unsweetened grape juice
SNACK	⅓ cup low-fat vanilla yogurt
LUNCH	2 oz. sliced turkey breast 2 slices whole wheat bread 2 tsp. diet margarine Lettuce and tomato slices Carrot sticks Apple
DINNER	3 oz. lean beef hamburger ⅓ cup mashed sweet potatoes flavored with 2 Tbs. orange juice ½ tsp. honey ½ cup orange juice

SNACK	½ cup Cheerios ½ cup low-fat milk Diced seasonal fresh fruits, ¾ cup

TUESDAY

BREAKFAST	3 Tbs. enriched Cream of Wheat cooked in water ½ cup low-fat milk ¼ cup mandarin orange slices
SNACK	Apple slices (½ apple)
LUNCH	1 cup chicken vegetable noodle soup with 2 oz. tofu slices added to soup 1 slice whole-wheat bread
SNACK	½ banana with ¼ cup low-fat plain yogurt (add 1 tsp. sugar if desired)

DINNER	2 oz. dry spaghetti cooked with
	    ½ cup tomato-meat sauce with
	    2 oz. lean meat drained of fat
	    ½ cup tomato puree, seasoned with
	    (onion and garlic powder, oregano)
	1 ear corn on the cob with
	    1 tsp. diet margarine
	1 cup cantaloupe and honeydew melon balls
	½ cup low-fat milk

WEDNESDAY

BREAKFAST	½ whole-wheat English muffin with 1 Tb. peanut butter 1 tsp. sugarless jelly ½ banana ½ cup low-fat milk

SNACK	oatmeal cookie ½ cup low-fat milk
LUNCH	Macaroni and cheese made with 1 cup noodles and 1 oz. American cheese ⅓ cup applesauce ½ cup low-fat milk
SNACK	1 uncoated frozen yogurt bar
DINNER	3 oz. broiled chicken (1 drumstick) 1 baked potato 2 Tbs. corn 1 oz. pumpernickel roll with 1 tsp. margarine ½ cup grape juice

THURSDAY

BREAKFAST	½ cup oatmeal 2 Tbs. raisins ½ cup low-fat milk
SNACK	1 slice whole-wheat bread 1 slice cheese
LUNCH	1 cup low-fat banana yogurt 2 graham crackers
SNACK	1 fruit-juice ice pop
DINNER	3 oz. broiled fillet of sole with 1 tsp. margarine 1 stalk steamed broccoli ⅓ cup brown rice ½ cup apple juice

FRIDAY

BREAKFAST	½ cup raisin bran ½ cup low-fat milk ½ sliced banana
SNACK	10 grapes
LUNCH	3 oz. tunafish in water, drained, with 1 Tb. diet mayonnaise 1 slice whole-wheat bread ½ cup low-fat milk ½ baked apple
SNACK	1 slice pumpernickel bread with 1 oz. cheese
DINNER	3 oz. meat loaf, lean and drained ¼ Tb. mashed potatoes made with low-fat milk 3 Tbs. green peas ½ cup low-fat milk

SATURDAY

BREAKFAST	½ orange, in sections ⅓ cup low-fat vanilla yogurt 1 tsp. wheat germ ½ pumpernickel bagel
SNACK	2 whole-wheat fig bars ½ cup low-fat milk

LUNCH	Egg salad sandwich made with
	    1 egg yolk (hard-boiled)
	    2 egg whites (hard-boiled)
	    1 Tb. diet mayonnaise
	    2 slices rye bread
	    Tomato slices
	½ cup unsweetened apple juice

SNACK	½ banana
DINNER	2 oz. cooked pot roast ⅓ cup carrots with 1 tsp. honey ½ cup noodles with 1 tsp. margarine ½ cup low-fat milk

SUNDAY

BREAKFAST	1 egg (scrambled) ½ whole-wheat English muffin ½ cup orange juice
SNACK	½ cinnamon-raisin bagel with 1 tsp. margarine
LUNCH	1 blueberry blintz, cooked in nonstick skillet 2 Tbs. low-fat plain yogurt ½ cup applesauce ½ cup grape juice
SNACK	2 rice cakes with 2 tsp. peanut butter
DINNER	1 cup chicken noodle soup 2 oz. sliced turkey breast 1 slice pumpernickel bread ½ cup fresh fruit salad ½ Tbs. Russian dressing ½ cup low-fat milk

# CHAPTER 21

Feeding the Over-Weight Preschooler: Just a Stage—or a Problem?

It is sad but true that many parents of fat children begin to look for a miracle at about the time their child reaches the age of four or five. These parents and their children are often the victims of two unfortunate myths. Myth No. 1 is that fat babies are healthier than thin ones. Believing the myth, these parents overfeed their infants and continue to overfeed them during toddlerhood. Myth No. 2 is that little children spontaneously shed their baby fat and begin to slim down during the preschool years.

I hope that we have already exploded myth no. 1. As far as losing "baby" fat goes, it just doesn't work that way. By about age three, food patterns that have been established earlier begin to solidify and unless parents intervene, the fat toddler grows into the fat preschooler. There will be no "spontaneous" slimming down. If your child is overweight, don't look for a miracle but rather look to *yourself*. Every month that you continue to allow her to eat more than she needs, every month that you neglect to instill good exercise habits, will allow your child to grow fatter, and the problem will become more difficult to deal with the longer you wait. The time to act is now. As far as fat-cell production is concerned, if your preschooler is fat, she will continue to multiply her fat cells at a rapid rate, and these greater-than-normal number of fat cells will stay with her for the rest of her life. Doctor Jerome Knittle, the fat-cell expert, has found that by age six some fat children already have more fat cells in their bodies than do many normal adults!

If your child is fat when she reaches the age of six, it is quite likely she will be fat at fifteen and thirty and beyond, especially if one or both of you, her parents, is also overweight. A recent study of 100 obese adolescents found that 45 of them had been overweight at six years of age. In another study, 85 percent of the fat adults who participated reported that they had been overweight at the age of five.

The problem is urgent, but the last thing I want for you is to become discouraged. As a matter of fact, if you can help your child stabilize her weight now when she is three or four or five, her chances of growing up at or near normal weight and staying there for the rest of her life will be much greater than if you wait for her to become a school-ager or adolescent before intervening.

If all this isn't enough to spur you into doing something about your preschooler's extra pounds, think about this: The longer you postpone action, the more likely she will grow up fat and suffer its consequences—namely, high blood pressure, heart disease, and certain types of cancer.

If you still need more convincing, remember that your preschooler will be starting first grade very soon. She will be meeting many new children, some of whom may be cruel enough to ridicule her about her weight. If she is clumsy as well as fat, which tends to be the rule and not the exception with obese children, she may be shunted to the sidelines by her schoolmates during games and team activities. The emotional consequences of overweight are painful and not easy to overcome, and your preschool-age child will surely face these consequences in the very near future if she remains fat.

Over the years I have treated large numbers of fat preschoolers. Based on my experience, the best approach is two-pronged:

1. Parents must provide their child with a diet that offers complete, well-balanced nutrition with somewhat fewer calories than she has been previously getting.

2. The mother and father must make sure that their preschooler becomes more active by planning and implementing a program of increased physical activity appropriate for her age and abilities.

With very few exceptions it is a mistake to put her on a strict, very low-calorie regimen, because such a diet may also be too low in the nutrients she needs for growth. The goal of the Eden Fitness Program for the fat preschooler is to slow down her too-rapid weight gain rather than to try to have her actually lose pounds.

Be prepared to have your will tested. If your child is too fat, it's a safe bet she got there honestly—that is, too many years of eating too much of the wrong foods and being less active than other kids her age. Though she is still young, she has already developed her own "lifestyle," complete with food preferences and fairly strong ideas about how active or how inactive she wants to be. She has learned that lifestyle from you. The foods she likes are the foods that you have given to her. If she overeats, it is either because you encouraged her or possibly allowed her to do so. If she sits around too much, again, it is probably because you have not urged her to do otherwise. It would be unrealistic to expect her to accept major changes in the way she exercises without complaining. You are going to have to be patient, firm, consistent, and unafraid to say "no."

In dealing with your overweight preschooler your "ace in the hole" may be her innate desire to emulate you. Remember, she wants to be more grown-up. And to her "grown-up" means being like mommy and daddy. I have worked with many, many parents who were able to harness their preschooler's natural desire to be just like them. In particular, I remember five-year-old Joey and his father. They looked almost exactly alike, both facially and in body type—both were markedly obese. The father had pretty much resigned himself to life as a fat person, but he could not accept the same fate for his son, and decided to take action. I explained the diet plus exercise approach and gave Joey's parents the Eden menu plans and food guidelines for preschoolers.

A few weeks later Joey's father called in desperation. "It's not working at all," he said. "Joey has been nagging and crying about food every day and we always end up giving him the wrong foods just to get a little peace and quiet in the house. There must be a better way." It took a bit of detective work on my part, but I discovered that Joey was being fed special foods and his parents were continuing to eat the same way they always had. I told this father that the only way to have any hope of success would be for him to join Joey on the same diet. He expressed doubts about how well it would work, because he had never been able to lose weight successfully, but he agreed to go along with my plan.

A month later Joey and his father entered my office, both beaming from ear to ear. "Me and *my* daddy are on the same diet," Joey informed me. "We are getting into shape together and will be *real* strong." The father winked at me. This particular story has a very happy ending. The program worked beautifully for both Joey and his father, and one year later both were healthier, more vigorous, and less obese.

Parental example is a powerful tool with the preschooler. If you appear to welcome and enjoy the vegetables, lean meat, fish, or chicken on your plate, chances are that your child will enjoy them also. If you don't eat the high-calorie, high-fat, high-sugar foods, she won't feel so "deprived" if you don't allow her to eat them. And if you don't buy, cook, or serve these foods, she can't eat them, at least not when she is at home (she probably will do much better visiting grandma).

This brings up the matter of "fat-proofing" your house. That involves going through the refrigerator, all the cabinets, and removing the bad stuff—the high-calorie, low-nutrition cookies and cakes and chips and drinks of various kinds. They're the No. 1 enemy when you are trying to help your child slim down. If you limit the bad stuff in your child's diet, see that she gets more exercise, try to set a good example in how you eat, and "fat-proof" the house, you will be able to bring your preschooler's weight under control. There will be times when you'll give in and allow her to eat something you know she should not have. When that happens, don't worry about it. If you stay on course most of the time, you will be doing fine. Even if you stay on course *some* of the time, your preschooler will be much better off than if you made no effort at all.

MEAL PLANS FOR OVERWEIGHT PRESCHOOLERS

MONDAY

The menus that follow were specifically designed for the overweight pre-schooler.

BREAKFAST	¾ cup orange juice
	Scrambled eggs (2 egg whites, 1 egg yolk, scrambled with
	   1 slice American cheese
	   ½ bagel
	   ½ tsp. soft margarine

LUNCH	Tunafish sandwich made with
	   3 oz. tuna in water, drained
	   2 slices whole-wheat bread
	   1 Tb. low-fat mayonnaise
	   Tomato slices and lettuce
	Grape juice soda made with
	   ⅔ cup grape juice
	   ⅓ cup seltzer

SNACK	1 cup skim milk 1 oatmeal raisin cookie
DINNER	4 ounces skinless chicken breast, steamed ½ cup broccoli florets ⅔ cup mashed potatoes with 2 Tbs. milk 1 cup fruit cup ½ cup skim milk
SNACK	½ cup ice milk

TUESDAY

BREAKFAST	¼ cup Wheatena cooked in ½ cup skim milk ¾ cup orange-cranberry juice
SNACK	Carrot-bran muffin ½ cup low-fat milk
LUNCH	2 slices whole-wheat bread 2 Tbs. peanut butter with 1 sliced banana 1 cup skim milk

DINNER	3 oz. oven-baked fish fillets with
	   1 slice (1 oz.) part-skim mozzarella cheese, melted
	   ¼ cup tomato sauce and
	   1 cup spaghetti
	   1 TB. grated Parmesan cheese
	1 cup green salad
	1 Tb. low-fat salad dressing
	½ cup skim milk

SNACK	¼ cup raisins

WEDNESDAY

BREAKFAST	½ cup whole-grain cold cereal ½ cup low-fat milk ½ banana ½ cup orange juice
SNACK	1 slice whole-wheat bread with 2 tsp. peanut butter ½ cup low-fat milk

LUNCH	Roast beef sandwich with
	    2 oz. lean roast beef on
	    pumpernickel bread
	    1 Tb. diet Russian dressing
	⅓ cup cole slaw, made with
	    diet mayonnaise
	1 fresh peach
	½ cup low-fat milk

SNACK	oatmeal cookie ½ cup low-fat milk

DINNER	1 slice pizza (6 oz.)
	Mixed green salad with
	    1 Tb. diet Italian dressing
	Sherbet float made with
	    ½ cup raspberry sherbet
	    ½ cup seltzer

SNACK	20 grapes

THURSDAY

BREAKFAST	1 poached egg 1 slice whole-wheat toast 1 tsp. diet margarine ½ cup orange-pineapple juice

LUNCH	Peanut butter and jelly sandwich
	    2 slices whole-wheat bread
	    2 Tbs. peanut butter
	    2 tsp. jelly
	½ sliced banana
	1 cup low-fat milk
	3 dried figs

SNACK	2 cups air-popped popcorn ½ cup low-fat milk

NUTRITION FOR THE OVERWEIGHT CHILD

DINNER	Spaghetti with meat sauce
	   1 cup spaghetti with
	   2 oz. chopped meat, drained of fat
	   ½ cup tomato sauce
	   Topped with 1 Tb. Parmesan cheese
	Carrot and celery sticks
	1 slice Italian bread with
	   1 tsp. diet margarine
	½ cup grape juice

SNACK	1 frozen juice bar

FRIDAY

BREAKFAST	½ cup low-fat vanilla yogurt 1 baked apple 1 Tb. wheat germ ½ cup cranberry juice Raisin bread with 1 tsp. margarine
LUNCH	1 cup chicken noodle soup 2 oz. tunafish packed in water, drained 1 slice rye bread 1 Tb. diet mayonnaise 1 slice watermelon 1 cup low-fat milk
SNACK	2 gingersnap cookies ½ cup low-fat milk

DINNER	3 oz. turkey breast
	1 medium sweet potato mashed with
	   1 tsp. diet margarine
	Tossed salad with
	   1 Tb. Italian dressing
	½ cup ice-milk
	Grape soda made with
	   ½ cup grape juice
	   ½ cup seltzer

SNACK	1 oz. peanuts 2 Tbs. raisins

SATURDAY

BREAKFAST	1 slice whole-wheat toast
	   1 Tb. peanut butter
	   1 tsp. honey
	1 cup low-fat cocoa
	½ banana

LUNCH	Apple or blueberry blintz, browned in
	   1 tsp. diet margarine, topped with
	   ¼ cup low-fat vanilla yogurt
	½ cup apple juice

SNACK	½ cup vanilla ice-milk

DINNER	Meat loaf made with
	   2 oz. lean hamburger meat
	   1 Tb. whole-wheat bread crumbs
	   1 Tb. grated Parmesan cheese
	   1 egg white
	2 small boiled potatoes
	¼ cup sliced carrots with
	   1 tsp. honey
	½ cup low-fat milk
	1 small bunch grapes

SNACK	1 slice whole-wheat bread with 1 oz. melted American cheese ½ cup apple juice

SUNDAY

BREAKFAST	⅓ cup low-fat cottage cheese ½ cup melon balls

	½ English muffin with 1 tsp. margarine ½ cup orange juice
SNACK	½ frozen banana coated with orange juice and wheat germ

LUNCH	Tuna melt with
	   1 slice rye bread
	   2 oz. tuna
	   ½ Tb. diet mayonnaise
	   1 oz. Swiss cheese
	½ cup low-fat milk
	1 apple, sliced

DINNER	Barbecued chicken
	   1 skinless chicken breast baked with
	   1 Tb. barbecue sauce
	½ cup broccoli
	1 pumpernickel-raisin roll
	   1 tsp. diet margarine
	¼ cup carrot salad made with
	   ¼ cup shredded carrots
	   2 Tbs. raisins
	   1 Tb. diet mayonnaise
	½ cup cranberry soda made with
	   ¼ cup cranberry juice
	   ¼ cup seltzer
	½ cup rice pudding made with
	   low-fat milk, brown rice, and honey

SNACK	Float with ½ cup vanilla ice-milk and ½ cup grape juice

CHAPTER 22
Meals for Overweight School-Agers

The emotional and psychological consequences of being fat during the school years can be especially painful. In this period, self-image begins to develop and it is important that a child perceive himself in a positive way. As self-awareness grows, however, the fat school-ager may begin to see himself as "different" because of his size and shape. To a child this age, "different" usually means "inferior." Other children begin to discriminate against him because of his weight. To make matters even worse, the parents who probably contributed to the problem by overfeeding him up to now, suddenly become critical. Whereas when he was younger, being fat was cute—now his parents no longer look at the extra fat the same way. This may be the cruelest cut of all.

I have never met a fat person of any age who would not instantly agree to become slim if that were possible. I have had heartbreaking conversations with hundreds of obese children who are miserable because of their weight. I remember what one ten year old told me when summarizing his weight problems this way: "My brother calls me two-ton. My parents continually nag at me. I have only one friend at school and she is heavy also." She had tears in her eyes.

In order to understand how a moderately reduced caloric intake plus increased caloric burn-off results in a significant weight loss, let us consider a hypothetical fat school-ager. If her parents plan meals that supply her with 250 fewer calories a day than before, she will have a calorie deficit of about 1,750 at the end of one week (250 × 7 – 1,750). Because there are 3,500 calories in a pound, that is the equivalent of ½ pound of fat. If at the same time she is encouraged to become more active and burns off an extra 250 calories a day in exercise, the caloric deficit at the end of a week will be 3,500—a whole pound of fat! Incidentally, a pound a week weight loss is a sensible, safe figure to shoot for.

That is how the calorie numbers work on paper, and that is how it would work for your child if you could monitor her every bite of food and direct her every action. We both know that in real life it just doesn't work that way. Your school-ager spends much of every day away from you in situations over which you have little control. Thus progress in losing weight may be much slower or at times nonexistent, but there will be some progress if you consistently exert your influence in the home.

Don't expect perfect cooperation from your child when you begin your efforts to slim her down. Although the meals and snacks you will be offering her are appealing and tasty (and there is enough of everything so that she will not feel hungry), and she'll have fun with the suggested physical activities and exercises, she is already set in her ways. If your child is fat, *you* must get her started on the path toward slimness and you must keep her going.

The first step always is to "fat-proof" your house. I have had experience with some parents who strongly object to this no junk-food-in-the-house policy, stating that if they follow it they will "deprive" a thin brother or sister or themselves for that matter. Not so. No one needs junk food, whether they're thin or fat. Everyone is better off without the enormous amounts of fat, sugar, and salt that these foods contain. In my opinion, ridding the house of foods that eventually contribute to a bunch of major health problems is a very *loving* thing to do for your family.

Let me tell you about the father who after listening to me talk at length about methods to help his daughter lose weight, suddenly jumped up and said, "Just a minute, Doctor. It sounds like you expect the whole family to make these changes."

"But of course," I answered. I thought he had understood this concept from the beginning, but obviously I was wrong. "We can't have Josephine eating fresh fruit for dessert when everybody else is eating chocolate cake, can we?" He did not bother to answer that question, but looked a bit depressed as he left the office. I wondered how successful Josephine would be in her weight-loss program. I must have gotten through, because things worked out very well for her.

If you are serious about wanting to help your child lose weight, you must accept that everyone in the family will have to eat pretty much as she does. This should not be a hardship. The foods that we recommend for her are healthy for everyone. The alternative—offering fattening foods to other family members while serving a lower-calorie diet to the fat child—is a blueprint for failure.

I would advise that you not make a big production about getting your school-ager to slim down. Sooner or later, probably sooner, you are going to have to explain to her that the foods that now appear on the table are different, why there are no cookies or cupcakes in the cabinets, why there are no sugary fruit drinks or soda pop in the refrigerator. What do you say? You simply state, "We don't eat those kinds of food anymore because they're not healthy"—PERIOD. Adding a few words about how this new way of eating will help to get her slimmer might be appropriate, but I would not belabor the point. You need not discuss calories with her or say that she should weigh herself frequently or tell her how awful it is to be fat. (She probably already knows that.)

Nor should you be super critical if, despite your explanations, she continues to ask and beg for candy and other junk food. In this context, criticism is never helpful; it will only make your child feel guilty and worthless, but won't stop her from still wanting the foods she's been used to eating. When you have to say no, say it as though you mean it and not as though your school-ager did a terrible thing in asking. In other words, skip the lectures. Don't scold. Don't nag. If you keep saying no calmly, firmly, but without blaming or accusing, she will begin to get the message.

Because your child (if she is fat) has probably been overeating all her life, don't expect a sudden about-face when you first begin to offer healthier, lower-calorie meals and snacks. After years of consuming too much of the wrong foods and, in effect, becoming addicted to them, she may now turn up her nose at the vegetables, fruits, lean meat, fish, and poultry that now appear on her plate. She may even believe that by refusing to eat these new foods she can get you to relent and give her the old-time foods. Don't fall for this not-so-subtle blackmail. Don't worry if she only picks at her food. Even if she misses a meal or two or three, no harm will come to her. I assure you, she won't starve. Most important, don't urge her to try to force her to eat. The urging you did in the past probably helped make her fat and so it's time to put a stop to it. Stick to your guns. Keep your house free of unhealthy foods and continue to make good wholesome foods available for snacks and at every meal. The interesting thing is that after a relatively short period of time your child will begin to eat and actually enjoy the Eden diet. Even if you don't believe a word of this, I urge you to give it a try anyway, and find out whether or not I'm right.

"What if Nancy gets junk food at a friend's house or stops off at the candy store after school?" a mother of a nine year old asked. This is a sensible question. You certainly should go on record and tell your youngster that you want her to keep those treats to a minimum. I don't believe that parents should constantly police or grill their children about what they eat when they're out with their friends. As I pointed out earlier, these outside eating experiences can slow weight loss progress, but in most cases the overweight child will lose weight over a period of months if her parents stick to the new rules of the Eden Fitness Program.

Some mothers and fathers have found that rewards help to keep their fat school-agers on the straight and narrow when they are out of the house. I object to the common practice of bribing children with food. It is *never* a good idea to offer a sugary "treat" if a child is "good." But a nonfood reward such as a record, a tape, something new to wear, tickets to a concert or sports event, and so on, is appropriate if the child has lost some weight. This reward system sometimes can make the difference between a child's giving in to junk food temptation or passing it by.

When your child has achieved the necessary weight loss and is now of normal weight, she can be switched from the diet for the overweight school-ager to the one for the normal-weight school-ager (see pages 00–00). Of course, bringing back junk foods into the house will without question result in your child quickly gaining back all her lost pounds.

MEAL PLANS FOR OVERWEIGHT SCHOOL-AGERS

Consult the following menus for help in slimming down your overweight school-ager.

MONDAY

BREAKFAST	1 cup raisin bran 1 cup skim milk 1 sliced banana

LUNCH	2 slices pizza made with English muffins
	   ½ cup tomato sauce or slices
	   2 oz. part-skim mozzarella cheese
	   1 Tb. Parmesan cheese
	Carrot sticks
	3 Tbs. raisins
	¾ cup unsweetened orange juice

DINNER	Chicken breast (skinless) baked with 1 Tb. Chinese duck sauce glaze ½ cup steamed string beans ½ cup brown rice ⅔ cup unsweetened apple juice Lettuce and tomato with 2 tsp. low-fat dressing

SNACK CHOICES	1 cup low-fat yogurt 2 cups air-popped popcorn ½ cup skim milk

TUESDAY

BREAKFAST	French toast made with
	    2 slices whole wheat bread dipped in
	    1 egg beaten with
	    2 Tbs. milk and ½ tsp. vanilla
	    1 Tb. syrup
	    1 tsp. diet margarine
	1 cup fresh fruit cup (strawberries, orange, melon)
	1 cup skim milk

LUNCH	Turkey sandwich made with
	    3 oz. sliced turkey breast
	    1 tsp. mustard
	    1 Tb. low-fat margarine
	    Lettuce, tomato
	    2 slices rye bread
	1 cup unsweetened apple juice

DINNER	2 cups cooked spaghetti with tomato sauce made with
	    1 cup crushed tomatoes
	    ½ cup mushrooms
	    ¼ cup green pepper
	    2 Tbs. onion, sautéed in
	    1 tsp. olive oil
	    2 Tbs. grated Parmesan cheese
	Tossed salad with lettuce, carrot, cucumber, and tomato with
	    1 Tb. low-fat salad dressing
	1 slice Italian bread
	½ cup skim milk

Meals for Overweight School-Agers 237

SNACK CHOICES	½ cup low-fat frozen yogurt

WEDNESDAY

BREAKFAST	Baked apple with
	   ⅓ cup cottage cheese and
	   2 Tbs. raisins
	1 cup low-fat milk

LUNCH	Peanut and butter sandwich
	   2 slices whole-wheat bread with
	   2 Tbs. peanut butter
	   2 tsp. unsweetened preserves
	½ cup fruit salad
	1 cup low-fat milk

DINNER	2 blintzes
	   1 cheese and 1 blueberry blintz
	   Fried in 2 tsp. margarine
	   Served with ½ cup low-fat vanilla yogurt
	1 bunch grapes
	1 cup apple juice

SNACK CHOICES	1 cup air-popped popcorn 1 cup grape juice 4 graham crackers 1 cup ice-milk

THURSDAY

BREAKFAST	1 cup cooked oatmeal made with
	   1 cup low-fat milk
	   1 tsp. margarine
	   2 Tbs. raisins
	1 cup orange juice

LUNCH	Macaroni and cheese made with
	   2 cups cooked macaroni
	   2 oz. shredded American cheese
	Tomato and cucumber slices with
	   1 Tb. Russian dressing
	2 oatmeal cookies
	½ cup low-fat milk

DINNER	4 oz. turkey breast
	1 medium baked sweet potato with
	   1 tsp. margarine
	   2 Tbs. low-fat plain yogurt
	½ cup steamed string beans
	1 uncoated frozen yogurt pop

SNACK CHOICES	1 small blueberry-bran muffin
	1 tsp. jelly
	Banana shake made with
	   ½ banana blended with
	   ½ cup low-fat milk
	   1 tsp. honey

FRIDAY

BREAKFAST	2 slices rye bread with
	   1 Tb. peanut butter
	   2 tsp. unsweetened jam
	1 sliced banana
	1 cup low-fat milk

LUNCH	Egg salad sandwich made with
	   2 hard boiled egg whites
	   1 egg yolk
	   1 Tb. diet mayonnaise
	   Lettuce and tomato slices
	   2 slices pumpernickel bread
	Carrot and celery sticks
	1 cup apple juice
	½ cup pineapple chunks

Meals for Overweight School-Agers

DINNER	Tuna and noodles made with
	    1 cup cooked noodles, mixed with
	    3 oz. drained tunafish and
	    3 Tbs. low-fat cottage cheese
	½ cup broccoli
	1 roll with
	    1 tsp. margarine
	1 cup strawberry ice-milk
	1 cup unsweetened grape juice

SNACK CHOICES	2 cups air-popped popcorn 2 fig cookie bars 1 cup low-fat milk

SATURDAY

BREAKFAST	1 slice whole-wheat toast with 1 slice melted American cheese ½ grapefruit in sections ½ cup low-fat milk

LUNCH	Turkey sandwich made with
	    3 oz. turkey breast with
	    1 Tb. regular mayonnaise
	    Sliced tomato
	    2 slices rye bread
	1 cup cranberry juice
	2 graham crackers

DINNER	1 cup hot and sour soup with 4 oz. tofu 4 salt-free Saltines Carrot and zucchini sticks 1 baked apple 1 cup grape juice
SNACK CHOICES	1 small bran muffin with 2 tsp. peanut butter 1 cup low-fat milk ½ cup rice pudding

SUNDAY

BREAKFAST
1 cup cooked farina made with
　1 cup low-fat milk
　1 tsp. margarine
　2 tsp. honey
1 orange

LUNCH
1 homemade pizza made with
　1 English muffin
　Toasted with 2 oz. melted mozzarella cheese
　¼ cup tomato sauce
Lettuce and carrot sticks
1 cup orange juice

DINNER
4 oz. baked flounder, stuffed with
　½ cup cooked spinach
1 baked potato with
　1 tsp. margarine
½ cup Grape-Nuts pudding made with
　low-fat milk
1 cup apple juice

SNACK CHOICES
2 oatmeal cookies
1 cup low-fat milk
½ cup strawberries

CHAPTER 23
Adolescent Obesity: What You Can Do About It

Parents of young adolescents often notice an increasing plumpness in their children, beginning at about the age of ten or eleven. "Is it just a stage she's going through or is she on the way to becoming fat?" they ask.

State or permanent condition? It's one of those questions for which the answer depends on several different factors. In many, maybe even most youngsters, there is an appreciable increase in subcutaneous fat during the year or so before puberty. It is almost as though the prepubescent body prepares itself for the coming adolescent growth spurt by storing a reserve supply of fuel. Thus in a sense, we can see that preadolescent plumpness is indeed a "stage." It is natural and fairly predictable.

This increase in subcutaneous fat isn't always temporary however. If a greater appetite without a corresponding increase in physical activity during these years leads to the manufacture of abnormally large numbers of fat cells, their numbers can never be reduced and so the child is stuck with them the rest of her life. The fat content of the cells will diminish if the adolescent loses weight, but the cells remain—always ready to fill up again with fat. The very presence of too many of these cells in the body makes weight gain easier and weight loss more difficult, not only during adolescence but for all the years that follow.

The overweight teen-ager already will have elevated blood cholesterol levels which, if allowed to continue to remain high, will become a definite risk factor for heart disease and stroke later on in life. But for the overweight adolescent, the health consequences of excess pounds are usually overshadowed by the emotional and psychological consequences.

Fourteen year olds don't worry too much about getting a heart attack many years in the future, but are very concerned about being well liked, being "one of the gang," being reasonably able to compete at sports, and meeting and relating with members of the opposite sex. Much as we adults might deplore the situation, the fat teen-ager is often perceived as being "different" and a "loser." Worse, that is the way she inevitably begins to see herself; this loss of self-esteem and positive body image causes grave psychological damage.

Overweight girls usually suffer more than boys, often becoming obsessed with the extra pounds and the feelings of inferiority and rejection that accompany them. Overweight boys, during the start of adolescence, may have a mental picture of themselves as being big and strong rather than fat. As time goes on, as the problem worsens and the mirror begins to reflect real obesity, these boys also start suffering.

I have never known a truly fat adolescent who was not inwardly miserable about her weight. This includes even the ones who have managed to convince their parents that they're happy and well-adjusted. When I get a chance to talk to these teen-agers without mama and papa in the room, the truth comes out. The truth is that they really want very badly to slim down.

You, the parents, can't lose weight for the fat adolescent, just as you can't get her a date for the prom or a place on the basketball team. You no longer have the tight control over what she eats, and the motivation for slimming down must now come from her. Remember that you have a more limited role to play than when she was younger. I don't mean to imply that there's no role at all for you in helping your teen-ager control her weight—she definitely needs your help. But the kind of help she needs most from you has little to do with demanding that she go on a strict diet. Rather, she must have cool, calm, unemotional support and *quiet* encouragement.

Most important of all, don't try to shame or embarrass her into losing weight. If she is fat, the shame and embarrassment are already acute. Her self-esteem is way down. Don't push it down further with harsh criticism of her appearance or eating habits. Successful weight control, like success in any other worthwhile endeavor, requires an initial confidence that the goal is somehow achievable. Without a certain measure of self-esteem, that kind of confidence is impossible.

An example of how not to behave was the mother of fourteen-year-old Carl, who literally dragged him into my office, sat him down in a chair, pointed a finger at him, and said: "Just look at that boy, Dr. Eden. Have you ever seen such a blimp? He is already wearing clothes four sizes larger than his father's! I tell him to go on a diet but does he listen? No! Tell me, what is the matter with him?" This outburst was very upsetting, both to me and to terribly embarrassed Carl. What made her outburst not only destructive but also ridiculous was that she was just as fat as her son.

Most parents are not as outspoken as this mother, but almost all experience anger, frustration, and guilt when their teen-agers are fat. They feel that it reflects badly on the way they have reared, disciplined, and influenced their child. They now start worrying about their teen-ager's health and happiness. So they often panic and become preoccupied and overinvolved with the problem. Unfortunately, all the anxiety about food on food makes the teen-ager more obsessed with eating, and thus less able to deal with the extra weight. A number of studies have clearly pointed out that there is an inverse relationship between the success rate of the treatment of adolescent obesity and the degree of parental involvement. In other words, the more involved the parents, the less likely their adolescent will be able to lose weight successfully.

This leads me directly to another important piece of advice for parents who want to see their teen-agers lose weight: Back off or better yet, *bug off*! Disengage yourself from the fray. If you have been playing policeman with regard to your child's diet, and if you have been keeping track of every bite when she's home and grilling her about what she eats when she's out, stop all that right now. Provide quiet support and encouragement. Let someone else, a doctor or trained health professional, supply the guidance.

To rule out any medical problems that might be affecting her weight, your child should have a complete physical checkup before attempting to slim down. Ideally, the doctor should be a pediatrician with plenty of experience in teen-age obesity. I would be suspicious of the physician who immediately prescribed pills or medication for weight loss. I am totally opposed to both these practices. I would also be suspicious of the doctor who did not seem sympathetic or particularly interested in working with your child or did not spend enough time discussing the problem. The doctor will probably want to confer privately with your adolescent, preferably at regular intervals. Let them work things out between themselves. Don't look for immediate dramatic results.

Another alternative would be to encourage your teen-ager to join a reputable weight reduction group (Weight Watchers and Diet Workshop to name two such organizations) whose programs are based on sound nutritional principles.

In dealing with the still-growing adolescent, it is important not to put the child on a diet that is too low in calories, because too rapid a weight loss might interfere with normal growth. Success is much better achieved simply by slowing down or stopping the rate of weight gain rather than trying to have the growing teen-ager lose weight too rapidly. To see how this might work, imagine a fourteen-year-old boy who is 5 feet one and weighs 160 pounds. Over the next couple of years with his adolescent growth spurt, this boy can be expected to grow four or more inches. If, through a modified diet and inceased physical activity, his weight can be kept steady at 160 pounds over that period, he will arrive at age sixteen only a few pounds above normal.

When obesity is extreme, especially if the teen-ager is almost fully grown, actual weight loss is desirable. But it must never be achieved through too drastic a caloric restriction or through the kind of fad diet where most of the calories come from just one or two food groups. Such diets are potentially hazardous for everyone, especially for growing youngsters. My rule of thumb is to tailor the weight-loss program in such a way that the fat teen-ager never loses more than 1 to 2 pounds per week.

It is a major mistake to beg, threaten, or nag your adolescent. The pressure to succeed, the motivation, must come from her. Nevertheless, it is still up to you to set up the circumstances that will make it easier for her to succeed. Family meals must be planned around healthy, nutritious foods that won't sabotage her efforts to control her weight. That means following the Eden diet guidelines. Lean meat, poultry, and fish, broiled or baked, never fried. Plenty of leafy greens and bright-colored vegetables. No elaborate sauces or gravies. No sugary desserts but instead, fresh fruit, low-fat cheese, or sugar-free Jello-O, not just for your overweight teen-ager, but for *all* family members.

You *can* make a difference. Through a supportive, encouraging attitude and the modifications you make in family meals and snacks, you can help your adolescent control her weight even though you can no longer completely control her diet. It requires patience and commitment, but the reward—better physical and emotional health for your child— is priceless.

During the many years that I have been treating obese adolescents I have come to realize that unless the teen-ager really wants to lose weight, the success rate is very low. I have developed a formula that has worked remarkably well for large numbers of fat adolescents, many of whom have previously tried and failed at diet after diet. The formula is simplicity itself, and if the teen-ager really wants to lose the weight, it is almost magical in its results. There are only two commitments that I ask from the overweight teen-ager, two iron-clad rules that they must follow:

1. Zero caloric intake from the end of dinner to the beginning of breakfast.
2. Thirty minutes of exercise *each day*, to be carried out anytime between the end of dinner and the beginning of

breakfast. This exercise can be anything from taking a brisk walk to swimming laps in a pool.

Obviously, these two commitments are in addition to the general guidelines of the Eden Fitness Program. Why has this formula been so successful? Because it combines a modest caloric restriction with increased caloric expenditure, and because it's so simple to follow. The properly motivated obese adolescent understands that these two commitments are a very small price to pay to lose weight and keep it off.

In analzying hundreds of food diaries that were faithfully kept by the overweight adolescents in my practice, it soon became obvious to me that most of them did an incredible amount of evening snacking with vast quantities of high-calorie junk foods. Simply by eliminating all the calories after dinner, the total daily calorie intake is often reduced by at least 500 calories (a single slice of plain cake with no icing has 360 calories; a glass of milk and a chocolate chip cookie have about 250 calories).

At the same time, 30 minutes of exercise each day burns off an additional 250 or so calories. A youngster who eliminates after-dinner snacks to the tune of 500 calories a day and burns off 250 calories more in exercise, ends up with a 5,250 calorie deficit in seven days, a 1½ pound loss in a week! It doesn't always work out so neatly, of course. A few adolescents lose more than that, especially at first. Others, usually the ones who eat more during the day to compensate for the snacks they won't have at night, lose less. The ones who choose a brisk walk for their 30 minutes of exercise don't do as well as those who choose swimming, bicycling, jogging, or working out on a rowing machine. But almost all make progress, and the heightened self-confidence that accompanies even modest success is enough to keep many of them on track.

I recently discussed this two-commitment program with fifteen-year-old Grace who was, conservatively, 40 pounds overweight. "But, Dr. Eden, going for a brisk walk for a half hour each night is much too boring. What else can I do?" I explained to her that she need not do the same kind of exercise each and every night. "Certain chores such as raking leaves or cleaning out the garage are also exercise. You could mow the lawn one day, for example, get in half an hour of ice skating the following day, and a half hour of walking the next. But somehow you must find a way to incorporate 30 minutes of using your muscles into each 24 hour period." She responded, "It sounds like a good idea, Dr. Eden, except for the fact that we don't have a garage or a lawn and there is no ice skating rink in our town."

We both got a good laugh out of this exchange. I am happy to report that Grace walked faithfully each night and in fact, lost her extra 40 pounds in six months.

FAT-PROOFING

"Fat-proofing" the house is a step you must take to help your obese adolescent lose weight. I have discussed this concept elsewhere in this book, but it is especially important when dealing with overweight teen-agers, because of their various appetites. By "fat-proofing," you eliminate all the junk food from your home, the trouble makers such as soda, instant drink mixes, cookies, cakes, potato chips, donuts, and other high-calorie, low-nutrition "baddies." If you can't bear to throw all that out, then give the stuff away. Don't keep a private reserve supply for yourself or for your normal-weight child. Your fat teen-ager will find it, I guarantee!

In place of the junk food, stock the refrigerator with a variety of fresh fruits and raw vegetables, low-fat yogurt, low-fat cheese, and unsweetened fruit juices. Be prepared for the complaints that will soon follow, such as "There's nothing decent to eat around here!" Simply smile, suggest one of the nutritious snacks stored in the refrigerator, and go about your business. The only explanation that you might give is that this is the way we eat around here because we are interested in everybody's health and well-being.

"What if she loads up on high-calorie foods when she's out of the house?" I can always count on being asked that question. The answer, of course, is that if she does eat too much of the wrong foods away from home, she won't be as successful at controlling her weight. Your child *knows* that. It is her choice to make and there is nothing you can do about it.

When parents do their part however—serve good nutritious, low-fat, low-sugar foods at family meals, and keep junk food out of the house—the overweight adolescent in those homes has a better chance of losing weight even though she continues to eat some of the bad stuff away from home. Believe me, it is worth your efforts.

Although details may vary from regimen to regimen, all the best and most effective weight control plans for adolescents allow for plenty of fruits and vegetables, servings of poultry, fish (more often than fatty red meat), moderate amounts of whole-grain bread and cereal products, and two or three glasses of skim milk daily.

MEAL PLANS FOR ADOLESCENTS

Four separate sets of Eden meal plans follow for the fat adolescent: (1) the growing overweight male teen-ager, (2) the growing overweight female teen-ager, (3) the fully grown overweight male teen-ager, and (4) the fully grown overweight female teen-ager. These meal plans have been carefully calculated to take into consideration the different caloric requirements of male and female teen-agers, as well as the different caloric requirements of the growing teen-ager and the fully grown teen-ager.

MEAL PLANS FOR THE GROWING MALE TEEN-AGER

MONDAY

BREAKFAST	1½ cups raisin bran 1 banana 1 cup of skim milk

	1 slice whole-wheat toast 1 tsp. margarine ½ cup orange juice
LUNCH	2 slices of pizza (plain) 1 cup apple juice

DINNER	1 cup oven-baked potatoes
	2 Tbs. catsup
	Meat loaf made with
	    4 oz. lean chopped meat drained of excess fat
	    1 egg white
	    2 Tbs. bread crumbs
	    2 tbs. chopped onions
	1 large tossed salad with
	    carrots, peppers, mushrooms
	    2 Tbs. low-fat dressing
	1 hard roll
	    1 tsp. margarine
	1 glass seltzer with cranberry juice

SNACK CHOICES	1 cup low-fat frozen yogurt with ½ cup sliced strawberries

TUESDAY

BREAKFAST	1½ cups Special K with ½ sliced banana 1 cup low-fat milk

LUNCH	1 cup minestrone soup
	4 saltines
	Grilled cheese and tomato sandwich
	    2 oz. cheese
	    2 slices rye bread
	    Sautéed in 2 tsp. diet margarine
	    1 Tb. mustard

½ cup grape juice mixed with
  ½ cup seltzer
2 whole-wheat fig cookies

DINNER

Chicken cacciatore
  2 pieces skinless chicken
  sautéed in ½ Tb. olive oil with
  1 cup mushrooms, onions, and peppers
  1 cup tomato sauce
Served on
  1½ cups cooked spaghetti
  1 slice Italian bread
  1 tsp. margarine
  ½ cup chocolate pudding made with
    low-fat milk
Seltzer

SNACK CHOICES

½ bagel with
  1 Tb. cream cheese
1 orange
1 frozen yogurt bar

WEDNESDAY

BREAKFAST

2 slices raisin toast with
  2 Tbs. cream cheese
  2 tsp. jelly
1 cup apple juice

LUNCH

Brisket sandwich made with
  4 oz. lean brisket
  Hard roll
  1 Tb. mayonnaise
Carrot and celery sticks
1 cup grape juice
2 oatmeal-raisin cookies

DINNER

6 oz. filet of sole stuffed with
  ½ cup spinach

Tossed salad with
  1 Tb. low-calorie salad dressing
1 large baked sweet potato
  1 tsp. margarine
1 baked apple
1 cup low-fat milk
1 slice whole-wheat bread

SNACK CHOICES
1 cup low-fat milk
1 frozen banana
½ English muffin
  1 slice mozzarella cheese
  ¼ cup tomato sauce

THURSDAY

BREAKFAST
Scrambled eggs made with
  2 egg whites
  1 egg yolk
1 English muffin with
  2 tsp. jelly
  1 tsp. margarine
1 cup orange juice

LUNCH
1 cup tomato soup made with
  low-fat milk
Chicken salad sandwich made with
  2 slices rye toast
  4 oz. chicken breast
  1 Tb. mayonnaise
Celery and carrot sticks
½ cup grape juice

DINNER
2 bean tortillas made with
  ¾ cup beans
  1 oz. shredded cheese
  shredded lettuce and tomato
  2 corn tortillas

	¾ cup rice 1 cup low-fat milk

SNACK CHOICES	2 whole-wheat fig cookies
	1 cup low-fat milk
	1 slice whole-wheat toast with
	  1 Tb. peanut butter
	  1 tsp. jelly
	1 cup low-fat milk

FRIDAY

BREAKFAST	1 cup raisin bran flakes ½ banana, sliced 1 cup low-fat milk 1 slice whole-wheat toast with 1 tsp. margarine

LUNCH	4 oz. hamburger
	  1 roll
	  1 Tb. catsup
	1 cup cranberry-apple juice
	1 orange

DINNER	1½ cups vegetarian chili made with
	  1 cup cooked kidney or pinto beans
	  2 Tbs. shredded cheddar cheese
	  1½ cups brown rice
	Tossed salad with
	  2 Tbs. dressing
	1 piece angel food cake
	1 cup low-fat milk

SNACK CHOICES	1 baked apple served with 1 Tb. maple syrup 1 cup low-fat strawberry yogurt

SATURDAY

BREAKFAST	1 cup orange juice
	1 cup cooked oatmeal made with
	   1 cup low-fat milk
	   3 Tbs. raisins
	   Sprinkled with wheat germ

LUNCH	Turkey sandwich
	   2 slices whole-wheat bread
	   4 oz. turkey breast
	   1 Tb. Russian dressing
	½ cup cole slaw
	Carrot and celery strips
	1 cup cranberry juice soda made with
	   ⅔ cup juice
	   ⅓ cup seltzer

DINNER	2 cups spaghetti
	¾ cup meat sauce made with
	   2 oz. chopped meat
	   ¾ cup tomato sauce
	   chopped onions, garlic, basil
	2 Tbs. Parmesan cheese
	1 slice Italian bread
	   1 pat margarine
	Tossed salad with carrot strips
	   1 Tb. Italian dressing

SNACK CHOICES	1 blueberry muffin 1 cup apple juice ½ cup ice-milk with ½ cup sliced strawberries

SUNDAY

BREAKFAST	2 whole-grain waffles, cooked
	   2 Tbs. maple syrup
	   1 tsp. soft margarine
	½ cup orange juice

LUNCH	Bagel with
	   4 oz. lean roast beef
	   2 tsp. mayonnaise
	   Lettuce and tomato
	1 cup grape soda made with
	   ½ cup grape juice
	   ½ cup seltzer
	1 banana

DINNER	6–8 oz. broiled fillet of sole with 1 tsp. margarine 1 cup brown rice 1 cup broccoli 1 slice Italian bread 1 cup low-fat milk 1 apple
SNACK CHOICES	1 cup ice-milk ½ cup blueberries

MEAL PLANS FOR THE GROWING FEMALE TEEN-AGER

MONDAY

BREAKFAST	1 bran muffin ½ grapefruit 1 cup skim milk
LUNCH	Egg salad sandwich made with 1 whole egg and 1 egg white, chopped

½ tsp. curry
1 stalk celery, chopped
1 Tb. diet mayonnaise
2 slices of whole-wheat bread
2 carrots, sliced
1 cup skim milk

DINNER

Chef's salad with
3 cups lettuce, tomatoes, carrots, cucumbers, mushrooms
2 oz. turkey breast
2 oz. lean ham
1 oz. cheese
2 Tbs. low-fat Russian dressing
1 rye roll
1 tsp. margarine
1 spritzer made with
½ cup cranberry juice
½ cup seltzer
1 uncoated frozen yogurt pop

SNACK CHOICES

1 orange
1 apple
1 oatmeal-raisin cookie
1 cup skim milk

TUESDAY

BREAKFAST

1 frozen waffle
2 Tbs. maple syrup
1 wedge honeydew melon
1 cup low-fat milk

LUNCH

Large baked potato stuffed with
⅓ cup low-fat cottage cheese
½ cup fresh, steamed vegetables, topped with
1 oz. part-skim melted mozzarella cheese
½ cup apple juice

DINNER	Chicken Hawaiian
	    4 oz. boneless chicken breast in cubes
	    1 cup diced pineapple
	    1 Tb. soy sauce, ginger, and garlic sautéed in
	    1 Tb. safflower oil
	¾ cup brown rice
	1 cup mixed vegetables, steamed
	Seltzer

SNACK CHOICES	1 oatmeal cookie 1 cup low-fat milk 1 small bag salt-free pretzels ½ cup low-fat lemon yogurt 2 dates

WEDNESDAY

BREAKFAST	1 cup Wheaties cereal 1 cup low-fat milk 1 sliced banana
LUNCH	1 slice pizza Tossed salad with 1 Tb. diet dressing 1 orange 1 cup low-fat milk

DINNER	Barbecued chicken
	    1 large skinless chicken breast
	    2 Tbs. barbecue sauce
	1 ear corn on the cob
	1 cup steamed broccoli
	1 pumpernickel roll
	    1 tsp. margarine
	1 cup grape juice

SNACK CHOICES	½ cup low-fat lemon yogurt 2 Tbs. raisins

1 slice raisin bread with
  1 Tb. cream cheese
1 cup low-fat milk
1 piece angel food cake

THURSDAY

BREAKFAST

⅓ cup low-fat cottage cheese
  1 cup diced pineapple
  1 Tb. wheat germ
  1 cup low-fat milk

LUNCH

Chicken salad sandwich
  4 oz. chicken breast
  1 Tb. mayonnaise
  2 slices rye bread
Celery and carrot sticks
1 baked apple
1 cup low-fat milk

DINNER

6 oz. broiled sole with
  1 Tb. mustard
  1 Tb. bread crumbs
1 cup steamed green beans
1 large baked potato with
  ½ Tb. each: sour cream and yogurt
Seltzer

SNACK CHOICES

1 cup ice-milk
½ cup sliced strawberries
2 rice cakes with
  2 tsp. peanut butter
½ cup rice pudding made with
  brown rice and low-fat milk

FRIDAY

BREAKFAST	1 cup farina 1 cup low-fat milk ½ cantaloupe

LUNCH	1 English muffin
	   2 slices melted cheese
	   ½ cup tomato sauce
	Carrot and zucchini sticks
	1 cup cranberry juice

DINNER	4 oz. broiled chicken 1 cup mashed potatoes with 1 tsp. margarine 1 cup steamed broccoli 1 whole-wheat roll 1 cup low-fat milk

SNACK CHOICES	1 frozen banana on a stick
	2 rice cakes with
	   2 tsp. fruit preserves
	   2 tsp. peanut butter
	1 orange
	½ cup low-fat lemon yogurt

SATURDAY

BREAKFAST	1 baked apple with
	   ½ cup low-fat vanilla yogurt
	   1 Tb. wheat germ
	½ cup orange juice

LUNCH	1 cup vegetable soup
	1 slice whole-wheat bread
	   1 oz. melted cheese
	   sliced tomatoes
	tossed salad with dressing
	1 cup low-fat milk

DINNER	2 cups spaghetti with 　3 oz. tunafish and 　2 Tbs. cottage cheese ½ cup carrots glazed with 　1 tsp. honey 1 slice raisin bread 　1 tsp. margarine 1 cup low-fat milk
SNACK CHOICES	1 pear ½ bagel with 1 Tb. cream cheese 3 cups air-popped popcorn 1 cup apple juice

SUNDAY

BREAKFAST	1 pancake with 　1 Tb. syrup 　1 tsp. diet margarine 　½ cup blueberries
LUNCH	Rice and beans made with 　¾ cup brown rice 　¾ cup refried beans made with 　½ Tb. oil 　Onions, peppers, and ¾ cup kidney or pinto beans 　2 Tbs. shredded cheese ½ cup corn 1 pear 1 cup low-fat milk
DINNER	4 oz. sliced turkey breast 1 cup mashed sweet potatoes 　1 tsp. margarine 1 cup steamed broccoli 1 cup low-fat milk 1 cup diced pineapple

SNACK CHOICES	2 rice cakes with 2 tsp. jelly 1 cup vegetable soup 2 saltines 1 uncoated frozen yogurt pop

MEAL PLANS FOR THE FULLY GROWN MALE TEEN-AGER

MONDAY

BREAKFAST	1 cup orange juice
	French toast made with
	    2 slices of whole-wheat bread
	    1 egg yolk
	    2 egg whites
	    2 Tbs. syrup

LUNCH	1 peanut butter and jelly sandwich with
	    2 slices whole-wheat bread
	    2 Tbs. peanut butter
	    2 Tbs. jelly
	1 cup skim milk

DINNER	2 lean pork chops, trimmed of fat and baked
	1 cup mashed potatoes made with
	    2 tsp. diet margarine
	    2 Tbs. milk
	1 cup glazed carrots with
	    1 tsp. orange marmalade
	½ cup applesauce
	1 milkshake with 1 cup ice-milk

SNACK CHOICES	½ cup low-fat vanilla yogurt ½ banana

TUESDAY

BREAKFAST	Bagel with
	    2 Tbs. cream cheese
	    1 cup orange juice

LUNCH	Brisket sandwich
	    4 oz. lean brisket
	    1 Tb. diet mayonnaise
	    Hard roll
	Carrot and celery sticks
	1 cup apple juice

DINNER	Red snapper, Greek style
	    6 oz. red snapper baked with
	    1 cup tomato sauce
	    1 oz. crumbled feta cheese
	    Oregano
	Tossed salad with
	    2 Tbs. diet dressing
	1 cup Spanish rice
	Baked apple a la mode, made with
	    1 baked apple
	    ½ cup ice-milk

SNACK CHOICES	1 cup low-fat vanilla yogurt with 3 Tbs. raisins and ½ oz. peanuts 2 oatmeal-raisin cookies 1 cup low-fat milk

WEDNESDAY

BREAKFAST	1½ cups Special K
	    1 sliced banana
	    1 cup low-fat milk
	1 slice rye toast with
	    1 tsp. diet margarine

262 NUTRITION FOR THE OVERWEIGHT CHILD

LUNCH	1 cup minestrone soup 4 oz. sliced turkey breast on hard roll with 1 Tb. Russian dressing Sliced tomatoes and carrots 1 cup apple juice

DINNER	Chicken cacciatore
	    2 pieces skinless chicken breast
	    Sautéed in 1 Tb. olive oil with
	        1½ cups mixed onions, peppers, and mushrooms
	    1 cup tomato sauce
	Served on 1½ cups spaghetti
	1 slice whole-wheat Italian bread
	    1 tsp. margarine
	½ cup chocolate pudding made with low-fat milk
	1 cup low-fat milk
	Tossed salad with
	    2 Tbs. diet dressing

SNACK CHOICES	½ cinnamon-raisin bagel with 1 Tb. cream cheese 1 cup orange juice 1 small bag salt-free pretzels 1 cup tomato juice

THURSDAY

BREAKFAST	1½ cups shredded wheat
	    ½ banana, sliced
	    1 cup low-fat milk
	½ cup orange juice

LUNCH	Grilled cheese and tomato, made in oven
	    2 slices rye bread
	    2 oz. Swiss cheese
	    Sliced tomatoes

	1 cup lentil soup 1 cup low-fat milk 1 apple, sliced

DINNER	Barbecued chicken
	    2 skinless chicken breasts
	    2 Tbs. barbecue sauce
	    1 Tb. Saucy Susan
	1½ ears corn on the cob
	Tossed salad
	    Lettuce, tomato, and cucumber
	    2 Tbs. diet salad dressing
	Cranberry spritzer
	    ½ cup seltzer
	    ½ cup cranberry juice
	1 piece angel food cake
	1 cup low-fat milk

SNACK CHOICES	1 low-fat strawberry yogurt 2 graham crackers 1 oz. peanuts mixed with 2 Tbs. raisins ½ cup grape juice

FRIDAY

BREAKFAST	1 cup orange juice 1 cup cooked oatmeal made with 1 cup low-fat milk 1 banana

LUNCH	Tunafish sandwich with
	    2 slices rye bread
	    4 oz. tunafish, packed in water
	    1 Tb. diet mayonnaise
	    Lettuce and tomato
	Carrot and celery strips
	1 pear
	1 cup low-fat milk

DINNER	2 cups cooked spaghetti
	¾ cup meat sauce made with
	  2 oz. chopped meat
	  ¾ cup tomato sauce
	  Chopped onions, garlic, and basil
	  Sautéed in 1 Tb. olive oil
	2 Tbs. Parmesan cheese
	1 slice Italian bread
	  1 pat diet margarine
	Tossed salad with
	  1 Tb. diet Italian dressing

SNACK CHOICES	1 bran-raisin muffin
	1 cup apple juice
	Cranberry float made with
	  ½ cup vanilla ice-milk
	  ½ cup cranberry juice

SATURDAY

BREAKFAST	2 whole-grain frozen waffles
	  2 Tbs. maple syrup
	  1 tsp. soft margarine
	½ cup orange juice

LUNCH	Bagel with
	  4 oz. turkey breast
	  1 Tb. Russian dressing
	½ cup cole slaw
	1 cup apple juice

DINNER	6–8 oz. broiled fillet of sole with
	  1 tsp. diet margarine,
	  lemon juice, and garlic
	1 ear corn on the cob with
	  1 tsp. diet margarine
	1 cup steamed broccoli with
	  1 tsp. sesame seeds

	1 whole-wheat roll with
	    1 tsp. diet margarine
	1 cup low-fat milk
	1 slice watermelon
	Tossed salad with
	    2 Tbs. diet dressing

SNACK CHOICES	1 cup ice-milk with
	    ½ cup fresh blueberries
	1 slice whole-wheat toast with
	    1 Tb. peanut butter
	1 cup low-fat milk
	1 cup vegetable soup
	4 salt-free saltines

SUNDAY

BREAKFAST	Scrambled eggs made with
	    2 egg whites and
	    1 egg yolk
	1 English muffin with
	    2 tsp. diet margarine
	1 cup orange juice

LUNCH	Peanut butter and jelly sandwich
	    2 Tbs. peanut butter
	    1 Tb. jelly
	    2 slices whole-wheat bread
	1 cup low-fat milk
	1 banana

DINNER	2 chicken tortillas made with
	    6 oz. shredded chicken breast
	    Sautéed onions and peppers in
	    ½ Tb. safflower oil
	    ½ oz. shredded cheddar cheese
	    Shredded lettuce and tomato
	    Rolled in 2 corn tortillas

	Topped with 2 Tbs. low-fat plain yogurt
	Served with 1 cup brown rice
	Grape spritzer made with
	½ cup grape juice
	½ cup seltzer
SNACK CHOICES	2 whole-wheat fig cookies
	1 cup low-fat milk
	1 slice rye bread with
	1 oz. melted cheese
	1 cup apple juice
	1 cup strawberry low-fat yogurt

MEAL PLANS FOR THE FULLY GROWN FEMALE TEEN-AGER

MONDAY

BREAKFAST	1 cracked-wheat waffle with
	½ cup sliced strawberries
	½ cup low-fat vanilla yogurt
	½ cup orange juice
LUNCH	1 cup spaghetti with
	½ cup tomato sauce with mushrooms
	2 Tbs. Parmesan cheese
	Grape juice float made with
	½ cup unsweetened grape juice
	½ cup seltzer
	½ cup vanilla ice-milk
DINNER	1 cup vegetarian vegetable soup
	Tuna melt with
	3 oz. tunafish packed in water, drained
	1 Tb. diet mayonnaise
	2 slices whole-wheat bread
	1 slice cheese

Adolescent Obesity: What You Can Do About It

	Lettuce, tomato slices 2 stalks celery 1 cup skim milk
SNACK CHOICES	2 cups air-popped popcorn ½ cup skim milk 1 oz. raisins

TUESDAY

BREAKFAST	1 small bran muffin with 1 Tb. apple butter

LUNCH	1 cup cooked noodles mixed with
	    3 oz. tunafish
	    2 Tbs. low-fat cottage cheese
	½ cup carrots, glazed with
	    1 tsp. orange marmalade
	1 cup low-fat milk
	2 fig bars

DINNER	Sweet-and-sour chicken
	    4 oz. boneless chicken breast baked with
	    2 Tbs. mustard
	    1 Tb. honey
	    1 Tb. soy sauce
	1 cup steamed green beans
	½ cup rice pilaf
	1 cup fresh fruit salad
	Cranberry spritzer made with
	    ½ cup cranberry juice
	    ½ cup seltzer

SNACK CHOICES	1 uncoated frozen yogurt pop ½ cup sliced strawberries topped with ¼ cup low-fat vanilla yogurt 2 graham crackers 1 cup vegetable soup 2 whole-wheat crackers

WEDNESDAY

BREAKFAST	⅓ cup low-fat cottage cheese with
	   1 cup sliced strawberries
	   1 Tb. wheat germ
	1 cup low-fat milk

LUNCH	Tunafish sandwich
	   3 oz. tuna
	   1 Tb. diet mayonnaise
	   2 slices pumpernickel bread
	Carrot and celery sticks
	1 pear
	1 cup low-fat milk

DINNER	4 oz. baked flounder made with
	   1 Tb. mustard
	   1 Tb. bread crumbs
	1 cup steamed broccoli
	1 medium baked potato with
	   2 Tbs. low-fat yogurt
	Seltzer

SNACK CHOICES	½ cup ice-milk with
	   ½ cup blueberries
	1 slice whole-wheat bread with
	   2 tsp. peanut butter
	½ cup vanilla pudding made with skim milk

THURSDAY

BREAKFAST	1 frozen waffle 1 Tb. maple syrup ¼ cantaloupe ½ cup low-fat milk

LUNCH	Grilled cheese sandwich, made in toaster oven
	    2 slices rye bread
	    2 oz. part-skim mozzarella cheese
	    Tomato slices
	½ glass apple juice

DINNER	Chicken cacciatore made with
	    4 oz. boneless chicken breast, in cubes
	    ½ Tb. safflower oil
	    ½ cup each: mushrooms, peppers, onions
	    ½ cup tomato sauce
	Served on ¾ cup brown rice
	1 cup steamed green beans
	1 small piece angel food cake
	½ cup low-fat milk

SNACK CHOICES	3 cups air-popped popcorn ½ cup low-fat vanilla yogurt with ½ sliced apple

FRIDAY

BREAKFAST	1 cup cooked farina 1 cup low-fat milk 1 orange

LUNCH	1 medium baked potato stuffed with
	    1 cup mixed steamed vegetables
	    ¼ cup low-fat cottage cheese
	    Topped with 1 oz. melted, shredded cheddar cheese
	½ cup low-fat milk

DINNER	4 oz. baked skinless chicken with
	    1 Tb. apricot glaze
	1 cup mashed potatoes made with
	    2 Tbs. low-fat milk
	    1 tsp. diet margarine

	1 cup steamed broccoli
	½ cup low-fat milk
	1 slice raisin-pumpernickel bread
SNACK CHOICES	1 frozen banana on a stick
	1 baked apple
	Cranberry float made with
	½ cup cranberry juice
	½ cup ice-milk

SATURDAY

BREAKFAST	1 poached egg
	1 slice whole-wheat bread
	1 tsp. jelly
	½ cup orange juice
LUNCH	1½ cups fresh fruit salad
	¾ cup low-fat cottage cheese
	Sprinkled with
	1 tb. wheat germ and cinnamon
	1 raisin-pumpernickel roll
	1 tsp. diet margarine
DINNER	Spaghetti with meat sauce
	1½ cups cooked spaghetti
	¾ cup tomato sauce made with
	2 oz.-lean, chopped meat
	Onions and peppers
	Sautéed in ½ Tb. olive oil
	2 Tbs. Parmesan cheese
	1 slice Italian bread
	1 tsp. diet margarine
	½ cup low-fat milk
	1 peach
SNACK CHOICES	1 oz. salt-free pretzels
	Strawberry shake made with
	½ cup low-fat milk
	½ cup strawberries

SUNDAY

BREAKFAST
1 pancake topped with
 ¼ cup low-fat vanilla yogurt
 ½ cup blueberries

LUNCH
Rice and beans
 ½ cup brown rice
 ¾ cup refried beans made with
 ¼ cup each onions and peppers
 ¾ cup cooked kidney or pinto beans
 Sautéed in ½ Tb. safflower oil
 Topped with 2 Tbs. shredded cheddar cheese
½ cup corn
1 apple
1 cup low-fat milk

DINNER
3 oz. sliced turkey breast
1 small mashed sweet potato with
 1 tsp. diet margarine
1 cup steamed broccoli
½ cup low-fat milk
1 cup diced pineapple

SNACK CHOICES
1 slice whole-wheat bread with
 2 tsp. honey
½ cup low-fat milk
1 cup vegetable soup
2 Saltines

Appendix

NUTRITION: THE BASICS

Nutrition is the food you eat and how the body uses it to live, grow, stay healthy, and to get energy for movement, warmth, work, and recreation.

Food is made up of different substances needed for growth and health. Food provides energy and nutrients that build and regulate the body.

Nutrients are substances essential to life that are present in food. The nutrients include carbohydrates, fat, protein, vitamins, minerals, and water.

THE NUTRIENTS

1. *Carbohydrates* are the simple sugars such as glucose (the sugar in blood), sucrose (table sugar), lactose (the sugar in milk); and the complex carbohydrates (or starch) found in flour, potatoes, bread, pasta, cereals, beans, etc.), which often contain dietary fiber (the indigestible portion of many fruits, vegetables, and grains).

Carbohydrates are the body's most efficient fuel and should supply more than half of all the calories we eat every day.

These carbohydrates calories should primarily come from starchy foods with fiber.

2. *Fats* include vegetable oils, which are liquid at room temperature, and butter, lard, and animal fats, which are solid at room temperature. Closely related to the fats are substances such as cholesterol and lecithin. Fats contain fatty acids that are either saturated, monosaturated, or polyunsaturated. The softer or more liquid a fat, the more unsaturated it is.

Foods that contain a large proportion of fat include well-marbled meats, oils, egg yolks, olives, butter, margarine, sour cream, whipped cream, ice cream, pie crust, and nuts.

Because the body easily makes fat from extra carbohydrate and protein that is eaten, it is not necessary to eat much fat. We need fat to provide us with the essential fatty acids that the body cannot make and which are supplied by polyunsaturated oils. We also need fat to aid in the absorption and circulation of many of the vitamins. Fats provide a concentrated source of energy, and act as insulation and protection for vital organs.

3. *Proteins* are food substances composed of amino acids joined together in a particular sequence that is unique to each protein molecule. The major sources of protein in the diet are meat, fish, chicken, eggs, skim milk, cheese, yogurt, soy and other beans, and nuts. Protein is used in the body to make and repair body parts such as skin, hair, nails, blood, bone, and muscle; and body chemicals such as enzymes, hormones, hemoglobin, and antibodies. Proteins also can be used to provide energy if not enough carbohydrates have been eaten.

4. *Vitamins* are small organic compounds present in foods, which are required by the body in trace amounts. They produce no energy but participate in a wide variety of metabolic processes. No one food contains all the vitamins needed by the body, so a diversified diet is important for an adequate intake of all the vitamins.

Vitamins are grouped into two categories: water-soluble and fat-soluble. Because water-soluble vitamins are excreted in the urine, they are rapidly depleted and must be replenished on a daily basis. Fat-soluble vitamins, on the other hand, are stored in fatty tissue and in the liver, and overdoses rather than deficiencies can be a problem.

5. *Minerals* are chemical elements that the body needs in trace amounts. Examples of some of the important minerals we need for good health include iron (Fe), calcium (Ca), Zinc (Zn), magnesium (Mg), and iodine (I).

Other important coneepts include:

Calories (kilocalories or kcal): The energy contained within food. One gram of protein or carbohydrate provides 4 calories, whereas 1 gram of fat provides 9 calories.

Fiber: The indigestible carbohydrate of grains, cereals, fruits, vegetables, and nuts, which contributes to the bulk of our diet. Fiber is also composed of soluble gums and pectins found in fruits and vegetables.

Cholesterol: A fatlike substance that is present in all animals as a structural component of cells, and as an important component of brain and nervous tissue. Cholesterol is used by the body for conversion to vitamin D and essential hormones such as aldosterone, estrogen, and testosterone, and the bile acids that enable us to digest fats. It is the main component of atherosclerotic plaque. In most cases, our bodies manufacture all the cholesterol we need, so we don't need to get cholesterol from our food.

Index

Accidents, 72, 174, 177
Acrobatic classes, 194
Adolescents, 124–61
 daily calories for, 52, 138, 248
 Eden diet plan for average, 138–61
 Eden diet plan for overweight, 241–71
 exercise for, 196–201, 241, 245–47
 helping overweight, 242–48
 iron needs of, 134–35
 meal plans for female, 145–50, 156–61, 254–60, 266–71
 meal plans for male, 140–45, 151–56, 248–54, 260–66
 parent's role in nutrition of, 128–31, 133–36
 rebellion of, 124–25, 134
 salt intake of, 136–37
 snacks for, 131–32, 138–39, 245, 246, 247
 sugar intake of, 135–36
 typical diet of, 126–27
Aerobic exercise, 46–47, 186, 194, 199–200
Allergies, 64
Allison, Dr. R. Curtis, 21–22
Allowance, 108, 115
American Academy of Pediatrics, 61, 63, 190
Amerian Cancer Society, 13, 95, 111
American Health Foundation, 12, 110
American Heart Association, 11–12, 95
American Journal of Diseases of Children, 31
Anemia, 30–32, 35, 37, 62, 68
Appendicitis, 39
Appetite, 91, 112–13, 207
 decrease in, 73–74, 75, 76, 210
 increase in, 126, 134, 241
 loss of, 32, 34

Arteries:
  plaque buildup, 4, 10, 13, 132, 274
  see also Atherosclerosis
Artificial food colorings, 53
Atherosclerosis, 4, 11–12, 13, 14, 16, 17, 274

Baking, 53, 245
Ball playing, 174, 180, 183
Beans, see Legumes
Beef, see Meats, red
Behavior problems,
  iron deficiency and, 31, 37
Betaendrophins, 45
Beverages, 97, 117
  see also specific beverages, e.g. Fruit juices; Milk; Water
Bicycle riding, 193
Bicycle Song, 182
Binging, 7, 212
Blackburn, Dr. George, 209
Blood pressure:
  exercise and, 45, 46, 47
  high, see Hypertension
Blue Bells, 168
Body image, 7, 242
Body type, 207
Botulism, 67
Bowling, 193
Brain, iron deficiency and the, 31, 32
Breads, 40, 53, 58, 67, 79, 96, 97, 106, 107, 115, 117, 130, 139, 248
Breakfast, 105, 106, 128–29
  menu guidelines, 54
  see also Meal plans
Breast cancer, 13, 51, 111, 133

Breast feeding, 60–62, 64, 69, 75–76
Breath-holding, 33
Broccoli, 113
Broiling, 53, 245
Brown fat, 208–209
Brown sugar, 25
  see also Sugar
Butter, 14, 16, 55, 56, 80, 109, 110, 273

Cake, see Junk foods; Snacks; Sugar
Calcium, 25, 34, 52, 113, 128
Calorie intake, 51, 52, 71, 88, 138, 248
  calorie-burning activities, table of, 212
  physical activity and, 179, 186, 189, 197, 210–13
Calories, defined, 274
Cancer, 4, 16–17, 205, 222
  diet and, 5, 13, 39–40, 51, 72, 80, 88, 93, 95, 104, 111, 116, 133, 201
Canned foods, 137
Carbohydrates, 213, 272, 273, 274
Carry-over sports, 47–48, 193–94, 200
Cavities, see Teeth
Cardiovascular disease, see Arteries; Heart disease
Cereals, 35–36, 40–41, 53, 75–76
  for infants, 64, 65, 66, 67, 68, 75–76
  iron-fortified, 75–76, 94, 96, 113, 128
  recommendations, 58, 79, 96, 106, 113, 139, 248

INDEX 277

Cheese, 53, 55–56, 58, 67, 80, 81, 113, 115, 130, 131, 133, 245, 247
Chicken, 52, 53, 56, 107, 110, 130
  see also Poultry
Cholesterol, 60, 71, 88, 93–94, 95, 109–11, 116, 126, 132–34, 273, 274
  daily intake of, 17, 51, 52
  foods high in fat and, 10, 14–15
  level of, in the blood, 4, 10, 12–13, 16, 45, 110, 205, 242
  lipoprotein factor, 13–14
Chores, 181, 187, 192, 194–95, 199, 212, 246–47
Cigarette smoking, 4, 16–17, 44, 111
Climbers, 181
Coconut oil, 14
Colon cancer, 13, 39–40, 51, 111, 133
Complex carbohydrates, 272
Condiments, 59
Constipation, 39, 40, 51
Cookies, *see* Junk foods; Snacks; Sugar
Cooking guidelines and tips, 52–53, 54–55, 79–80, 116
Crawling games, 180
Creeping by infants, 166, 170
Crib devices, 166
Crosby, Dr. William, 210
Cured meats, 80, 96

Dairy products, *see individual products, e.g.* Butter; Eggs; Milk

Dancing, 182, 185, 186, 194, 200
Deep frying, *see* Fried foods
Delicatessen meats, 80, 96
Dental care, *see* Teeth
Depression, 7, 45
Diabetes, 40, 51, 111
Diet, *see* Eden diet plan; *specific foods and nutrients*
Dinner, 105, 108–109, 130
  menu guidelines, 54
  snacks after, 245, 246
  see also Meal plans
Diverticulitis, 39, 51
Diverticulosis, 51
DNA synthesis, 32
Dover, 175
Dyment, Dr. Paul, 190

Ectomorphs, 207
Eden diet plan:
  for adolescents, 138–61, 241–71
  cooking tips, 52–53, 54–55, 79–80, 115
  fats and cholesterol intake on, 17, 51, 52, 53
  fiber intake on, 51, 52, 53
  general recommendations, 52–53, 54–59
  goals of, 51
  guidelines for menu planning, 54
  for infants, 60–69
  iron intake on, 51, 52
  for overweight children, 77–78, 214–71
  for preschoolers, 95–102
  salt intake on, 22, 51, 52, 53
  for school-age children, 116–23, 231–40

278 INDEX

Eden diet plan: *(continued)*
  sugar intake on, 28–29, 52, 53
  for toddlers, 79–86, 214–20
Eden exercise plan, *see* Exercise
Eggs, 16, 53, 55, 65, 67, 80, 96, 107, 109, 110, 130, 133
Emotional consequences of obesity, 205, 215, 222, 231, 242–43
Endomorphs, 207
Erasmus University Medical school, 21
Exercise, 6–7, 43–48, 103, 104, 165–201
  for adolescents, 196–201, 241, 245–47
  aerobic, 46–47, 186, 194, 199–200
  calorie-burning activities, table of, 212
  carry-over sports, 47–48, 193–94, 200
  fat metabolism and, 208–209, 211
  health benefits of, 17, 44–46, 194–98
  for infants, 165–76
  insufficient, 4, 6–7, 43–44, 111, 170–71, 174, 178–79, 184, 185, 186, 189–92, 195, 196, 199, 201, 210–11, 212
  for preschoolers, 184–88, 221, 223
  prevention of obesity and, 209–12
  for school-age child, 189–95
  setting an example, 44, 191–92, 198
  sodium pump efficiency and, 209
  for toddlers, 177–83

Fad diets, 245
Family outings, 186, 194
Fat (body), 206–207, 208, 210–11
  development of fat cells, 214–15, 221–22, 241
  types of, 208
Fats (dietary), 10–17, 40, 51, 52, 53, 54, 55, 71, 80, 88, 93–94, 109–11, 116, 126, 127, 132–34, 213, 273
Fatty acids, long-chain, 14
Fiber, 39–42, 51, 52, 88, 111, 116, 126, 272, 274
Fish, 14, 52, 53, 56, 80, 96, 107, 110, 130, 133, 245, 248
Fluoride, 27, 63
Folic acid, 40
Fomon, Dr. Samuel, 64
Formula, commercial, 61, 62, 67, 68, 69, 75–76
Four-wheeled vehicles, 181
Franks, Dr. Bert M., 197
Fried foods, 53, 54, 55, 80, 109, 110, 245
Frozen goodies as snacks, 97, 139
Fructose, 25
Fruit juices, 34, 36
  in infant bottle, 66
  limiting, 112–13
  recommendations, 57, 80, 96, 97, 106, 107, 128, 131, 247

Fruits, 40, 41, 52, 57, 58, 67, 80, 96, 106, 107, 111, 114, 115, 117, 128, 130, 131, 138, 245, 247, 248
  dried, 35, 36, 58, 134, 138

Gastrointestinal
  diseases, 39–40, 51
Genetics and obesity, 206–207
Glucose, 272
Goldring, Dr. D., 46
Grad Open, Shut Them, 188
Grains, 40–42, 53, 58, 67, 111, 115, 128, 139, 248
Gravies, 245
Growth, 32, 48, 73–74
Gymboree®, 167, 181
Gymnastics, 186, 194

Harvard Medical School, 209
  Children's Medical Center at, 22
Head and Shoulders, 181
Heart, 46, 47, 197, 208
Heart attack, 10, 12, 16, 19, 20, 45, 46, 51, 72, 93, 95, 116, 132, 133, 136, 184, 189, 197, 201
  risk factors, 110–11, 205
Heart disease, 4, 222, 242
  diet and, 5, 11–13, 16, 27, 40, 88, 104
Heart Lung and Blood Institute, 12
Hematocrit levels, 32
Hemoglobin, 31, 32
Herbs, 59, 115
Hersch, Dr. Jules, 210
High blood pressure, *see* Hypertension
High-denisty lipoprotein (HDL), 13–14, 45

Hiking, 186
Hofman, Dr. Albert, 21
Honey, 25, 66–67
Honey Industry Council of America, Inc., 67
Honig, Dr., 33
Hop and skip games, 180
Hunemann, Dr. Ruth L., 211
Hyperactivity, 26
Hypertension, 4, 46, 51, 205, 222
  diet and, 5, 20–22, 72, 88, 95, 116, 136–37
  diseases linked to, 20
  exercise and, 45, 46–47, 184, 189–90, 197, 201
Hypothalmus, 207

Ice cream, 14, 53, 56, 58
Ice milk, 56, 58, 81, 139
Immune system, 32
Infants, 60–69
  breast feeding, 60–62, 64, 69, 75–76
  common feeding mistakes, 60
  exercise for, 165–76
  fat, 68–69
  fluoride for, 63
  introducing solid foods, 60, 63–68
  overfeeding, 60, 61–62
  salt and sugar in diet of, 60, 62, 66–67
  switching to cow's milk, 60, 62, 68, 75–76
IQ scores, 34
Iron, 25, 30–38, 71, 88, 116, 126
  absorption, 36
  deficiency, 30–38, 51, 60, 61, 62, 68, 75–76, 94–95, 111–14

INDEX

Iron *(continued)*
  foods fortified with, 61, 66, 75–76, 94–95, 96, 113, 128
  foods rich in, 35–36, 68, 94–95, 112, 134–35
  on menu plans, 52
  supplements, 37–38, 94–95
Irritability, 32, 51

Japan, 20, 132–33
Jello-O, sugar-free, 245
Jobs, part-time, 199
Jogging, 186, 198, 200
Johns Hopkins School of Medicine, 31
Jollife, Dr. Norman, 207
Journal of the American Medical Association, 21, 210
Jumping rope, 193, 200
Junk foods, 73, 88–93, 105, 108, 114–15, 125, 127, 130, 131–32, 212–13, 235, 246, 247
  "fat-proofing" your house, 224, 232, 247–48
Just Like Me, 171

Kallahari Bushmen, 20
Kicking toys, 166
Kidney problems, 60, 62, 136
  failure to function, 19, 20
Knittle, Dr. Jerome L., 214, 215, 222

Lactose, 25, 272
Lamb, 52, 56, 80, 133
  see also Meats, red
Lauer, Dr. Ronald, 11
Lead poisoning, 76
Learning problems, iron deficiency and, 31, 33–34, 37, 51, 68, 94–95, 112
Lecithin, 273
Leg exercises, 165–66
Legumes, 40, 41, 53, 58, 67, 80, 133, 134
Levy, Dr. Robert, 12
Lipoproteins, 13–14, 45
Liver, 34, 35, 134
Los Angeles Pediatric Society, 21
Love Is A Circle, 169
Low-density lipoprotein (LDL), 13–14
Lunch, 105, 129–30
  menu guidelines, 54
  packing your child's, 105, 107, 129–30
  see also Meal plans
Lungs, 46, 47, 197

Margarine, 55–56, 109
Mayer, Dr. Jean, 210–11
Mayonnaise, 55, 56
Meal plans:
  for adolescents, 140–61, 248–71
  guidelines for each meal, 54
  for preschoolers, 97–102, 225–30
  for school-age children, 118–23, 235–40
  for toddlers, 82–86, 216–20
Meats, 52, 53, 56
  fish, *see* Fish
  poultry, *see* Poultry
  recommendations, 67, 80, 96, 110, 130, 245, 248
  red, 10, 13, 14, 35, 52, 56, 80, 96, 107, 109, 110, 133, 248

Meats *(continued)*
  smoked, cured, and salted, 80, 96, 137
Menstruation, 134
Menus, *see* Meal plans
Metabolism, 32, 208–209, 210, 213
Milk (breast), *see* Breast feeding
Milk (cow's), 55–56, 69
  limiting amount of, 34, 80, 96, 112–13
  puddings, 139
  skimmed and low-fat, 53, 55–56, 69, 80, 81, 96, 106, 107, 110, 113, 115, 128, 130, 133, 248
  switching infant to, 60, 62, 68, 75
  whole, 10, 13, 53, 56, 109, 110, 113, 133
Minerals, 274
  supplements, *see* Vitamin supplements
  supplied on menu plans, 52
  see also individual minerals
Molasses, 25
Monosaturated fats, 273
Morgan, Dr. Beverly, 21
Mt. Sinai Medical Center, 214
Moving, 175–76
Multivitamins, *see* Vitamin supplements
Myocardial infarction, *see* Heart attack

National Cancer Institute, 39–40
National Institutes of Health, 16, 110
Neck muscles, infant's, 165
Newman, H. H., 207
Nitrates, 53

Nitrites, 53, 80
Nonstick cookware, 55
Nutrients, 272–74
  see also individual nutrients
Nutritional density, 25
Nuts, 41, 58

Obese children, 205–71
  adolescents, 241–71
  adult obesity and, 68, 72, 95, 205–206, 213, 222
  daily calories for, 52, 248
  eating patterns of, 212–13
  Eden diet plans for, 78, 214–71
  exercise factors, 209–12
  genetic factors, 206–207
  health dangers for, 205
  metabolic factors, 208–209, 210, 213
  preschoolers, 221–30
  school-age, 231–40
  toddlers, 214–20
  see also Obesity
Obesity, 4, 7, 17, 45, 51, 60, 88, 104, 170
  calorie balance and, 206
  childhood, and adult, 68–69, 72, 95, 205–206, 213, 222
  diseases linked to, 111, 205, 222
  physical inactivity and, 179, 189–90, 197
  sugar intake and, 26, 136
  see also Obese children
Oils, 53, 55
  vegetable, 14, 16, 56, 59, 273
Oski, Dr. Frank, 31, 33
Osteoporosis, 51
Overfeeding, 60, 61–62, 64

INDEX

Overprotectiveness, 174, 177–78

Palm oil, 14
Passani, Dr. Eugene, 16
Pasta, 55, 58, 67
Peanut butter, 58, 80, 107, 130, 133
Peas, *see* Legumes
Pediatrician, 71, 244
Pediatric News, 197
Peer games, 187
Physical checkup, 244
Pica, 33, 76
Pickled foods, 137
Play Arena, 167
Play yard, outdoor, 180–81, 186
Poaching, 53
Pollitt, E., 113
Polyunsaturated fats, 14, 16, 273
Popcorn, 58
Pork, 52, 56, 80, 133
   see also Meats, red
Position for carrying infant, 165
Potassium, 209
Potatoes, 58, 80
Poultry, 56, 80, 96, 133, 245, 248
   see also Chicken
Preschoolers, 87–102
   cholesterol and fat intake of, 93–94
   daily calories for, 52
   Eden diet plan for average, 95–102
   Eden diet plan for overweight, 221–30
   establishing good eating habits for, 88–93, 222–25
   exercise for, 184–88, 223
   iron needs of, 95
   meal plans for, 97–102, 225–30
   personality of, 87–88, 223–24
   setting an example for, 223–24
   snacks for, 96–97, 224
President's Council on Physical Fitness, 7, 44
Preventive medicine, 16, 21–22
Prostate cancer, 13, 111
Protein, 62, 128, 213, 273, 274
   recommendations, 80, 133
Push and pull toys, 180, 182
Push-ups, 172
Psychological benefits of exercise, 197–98
Puddings, 139

Qush' kua nomads, 21

Rectum, cancer of the, 39–40
Red blood cells, 31
Respiratory infections, 72
Rice, *see* Pasta
Right Hand, Left Hand, 182
Rockefeller University, 210
Rocking by infants, 166, 170
Roly Poly, 167–68
Rope jumping, 193, 200
Roughhousing, 180, 186–87
Row, Row, Row, Your Boat, 175
Row Your Boat, 187
Running, 182, 184, 200

Salad dressing, 55, 59
Salads, 53
Salt, 51, 59, 60, 71, 73, 88, 126, 127, 128, 136–37, 138

Salt *(continued)*
  avoiding child's acquiring a taste for, 22, 66
  foods high in, 18, 19–20, 59, 62, 69
  hypertension and, 20–22, 136–37
  on menu plans, 52
  salted meats, 80, 96, 137
  ways to limit intake of, 53, 55, 96, 115, 137
Saturated fats, 11, 14, 16, 17, 40, 80, 93–94, 132, 273
Sauces, 55, 59, 245
Sautéing, 55
Schneiderman, Dr. Marvin, 39–40
School-age children, 103–23
  breakfast for, 105, 106
  daily calories for, 52
  dinner for, 105, 108–109
  Eden diet plan for average, 116–23, 235
  Eden diet plan for overweight, 231–40
  exercise for, 189–95
  fat and cholesterol intake of, 109–11
  independence of, 103–106
  iron deficiency in, 111–14
  lunch for, 105
  meal plans for, 118–23, 235–40
  salt intake of, 115, 116
  snacks for, 105, 107–108, 114–15, 116–17, 232, 233, 234
  sugar intake of, 114–15
Seeds, 41, 59
Self-esteem, 197, 231, 242, 243, 246
Seshadri, Dr. S., 33–34
Seventh Day Adventists, 133
Shortening, vegetable, 14
Skating, 193, 198, 200
Skip and hop games, 180
Slides, 181
Smoked meats, 80, 96, 137
Smoking, *see* Cigarette smoking
Snacks, 212–13
  for adolescents, 131–32, 138–39, 245, 246, 247
  after dinner, 245, 246
  caloric value of popular, 213
  "fat-proofing" your house, 224, 232, 247–48
  menu guidelines, 54
  for preschoolers, 96–97, 224
  recommended, 58
  for school-age children, 105, 107–108, 113–14, 116–17, 232, 234
  for toddlers, 73, 74, 75, 81
Soccer, 183, 187, 194
Soda, 96, 106, 107, 114
Sodium, *see* Salt
Sodium-potassium pump, 209
Soft drinks, *see* Soda
Solid foods, introduction of, 60, 63–68
Sour cream, 55
Space Mountain, 176
Spices, 59, 115
Spinach, 112
Sports, 193–94, 200–201
  carry-over, 47–48, 193, 200
Standing by infants, 166–67
Stir-frying, 55
Stretch, Stretch, 181
Stroke, 4, 19, 20

Stroke *(continued)*
  diet and, 5, 16, 20, 27, 51, 88, 93, 95, 104, 116, 132, 136
  exercise and, 45, 46, 184, 189, 197, 201
  risk factors, 111, 205, 242
Sucrose, 25, 272
Sugar, 23–29, 60, 71, 73, 88, 89, 96, 126, 128, 129, 135–36, 272
  associations with foods high in, 24, 93
  craving for, 23–24, 25–26, 66, 135–36, 213
  cutting down on, 27–29, 114–15, 136, 245
  health problems related to, 26–27
  lack of nutritional value, 25, 74, 212–13
  level of, in the blood, 40
  on menu plans, 52
  setting an example, 28
  toddler's demands for, 72–73
Sway, Sway II, 171
Sweets, *see* Junk foods; Snacks; Sugar
Swimming, 182–83, 185, 186, 193, 198, 200

Teenagers, *see* Adolescents
Teeth:
  fluoride for, 27, 63
  sugar consumption and, 26–27
Television, 178, 185, 189, 190, 191, 199
  workout shows, 194, 199
Television advertising, 89
Tennis, 193, 200

Texas Christian University Health Center, 197
Toddlers, 70–86
  control over diet of, 76–78
  daily calories for, 52
  decrease in appetite, 74–75, 76
  Eden diet plan for average, 79–86
  Eden diet plan for overweight, 214–20
  exercise for, 177–83, 215, 216
  giving in to demands of, 72–73
  great food wars stage, 73–74
  iron deficiency in, 75–76
  meal plans for, 82–86, 216–20
  setting an example, 78
  snacks for, 75, 81
  wrong foods in diet of, 71–72
Tricycles, 182
Turkey, 52, 56
  see also Poultry
Turn-over games, infant, 166
Turn, Turn, Turn Around, 170
Twins: A Study of Heredity and Environment (Newman), 206–207

U.S. Center for Disease Control, 67
U.S. Department of Agriculture, 23
U.S. Department of Health and Human Services, 43, 190, 196
University of California, 21, 211
University of Iowa School of Medicine, Division of Pediatric Cardiology, 11

Veal, 56, 80, 96, 133
Vegetable oils, 14, 16, 56, 58, 59, 273
Vegetables, 40, 41, 42, 53, 57, 58, 67, 77, 78, 79, 80, 96, 107, 111, 115, 117, 130, 131, 139, 245, 247, 248
  leafy green, 34, 35, 94, 134, 245
Vehicles, riding, 181, 182
Video workouts, 194
Vitamin A, 40
Vitamin C, 36, 40, 52
Vitamins, 116, 128, 273–74
  supplied on menu plans, 52
Vitamin supplements, 38, 63, 68, 76, 94, 114

Walking, 173–74, 187, 198, 199, 200, 246, 247

Water, 34–35, 66, 112
Wayne State University, School of Medicine, 210
Weight reduction, 46, 241, 243–45
  regaining lost weight, 206, 214–15, 235
  rewarding, 234–35
  see also Obese children; Obesity
Weight reduction groups, 244
Wheels on the Bus, 168–69
Whipped cream, 53
Wrestling, 183, 186

X Marks the Spot, 172

Yeah-Yeah, 173
Yellow fat, 208–209
Yogurt, 55, 56, 58, 67, 80, 81, 113, 115, 131, 133, 247

① SIGNET (0451)

FOR THE PARENT-TO-BE

☐ **PAMPERS PARENTS' HANDBOOK by Alvin N. Eden, M.D.** The essential parenting guide, written by an eminent pediatrician, that answers all the urgent questions parents ask during the first year of their baby's life. This easy-to-read book provides you with invaluable advice on choosing your baby's doctor, what to do when the baby won't stop crying, how to prevent diaper rash, how to help your baby sleep through the night, and much more. (148282—$3.95)

☐ **PREPARATION FOR CHILDBIRTH: A Lamaze Guide by Donna and Rodger Ewy.** Here is the book to instruct prospective parents in the Lamaze techniques for easier childbirth, complete with diagrams and photographs outlining each sequence from labor through delivery. "Excellent ... provides the necessary tools for a self-controlled, shared childbirth experience."—*The Bookmark* (158938—$4.95)

☐ **PREGNANCY, BIRTH, AND FAMILY PLANNING by Alan F. Guggmacher, M.D. Revised and updated by Irwin H. Kaiser, M.D.** This famous book tells you all you want and need to know about having a baby, in terms that everyone can understand. Including the latest developments in medical technology and practice, it is arranged for easy reference in time of need. By explaining carefully and completely what lies ahead at each stage of pregnancy and birth, this book makes child-bearing the worry-free and joyfully fulfilling experience that it can and should be. (147626—$4.95)

☐ **SOLO PARENTING: YOUR ESSENTIAL GUIDE** *How to Find the Balance Between Parenthood & Personhood* **by Kathleen McCoy.** In this comprehensive sourcebook, the author talks with over one hundred solo parents, as well as dozens of professionals, and offers ideas for coping with the tough issues facing single parents. Listings of counseling services, hotline and support organizations. (151372—$4.50)

Prices slightly higher in Canada

Buy them at your local bookstore or use this convenient coupon for ordering.

NEW AMERICAN LIBRARY
P.O. Box 999, Bergenfield, New Jersey 07621

Please send me the books I have checked above. I am enclosing $_____
(please add $1.00 to this order to cover postage and handling). Send check or money order—no cash or C.O.D.'s. Prices and numbers are subject to change without notice.

Name_____

Address_____

City _____ State _____ Zip Code _____

Allow 4-6 weeks for delivery.
This offer is subject to withdrawal without notice.

⓪ SIGNET (0451)

BRINGING UP BABY

☐ **HOW TO DISCIPLINE WITH LOVE: From Crib to College by Dr. Fitzhugh Dodson.** A leading authority on child-rearing offers parents a flexible program of positive reinforcement for teaching children desirable behavior at every stage of development. (159063—$4.95)

☐ **HOW TO FATHER by Dr. Fitzhugh Dodson.** An authority on child care guides the new father through all stages of child's growth—from infancy through adolescence—instructing him on discipline, teaching, affecting his child's moods, developing his interests, and forming a loving and positive child-father relationship. Appendices, illustrations and Index included. (154363—$4.95)

☐ **HOW TO PARENT by Dr. Fitzhugh Dodson.** Based on a common sense combination of love and discipline, Dr. Dodson's approach to child-raising offers a creative, complete, and mutually enjoyable program for helping parents guide their children through the all-important years from birth to five. (156250—$4.95)

☐ **HOW TO REALLY LOVE YOUR CHILD by Ross Campbell, M.D.** This famed psychiatrist who has helped countless parents with "problem children" tells how to successfully communicate your love for your child even in times of stress and when discipline is necessary. Clearly written, with a wealth of case histories. (153464—$3.50)

☐ **DR. MOM: A Guide to Baby and Child Care by Marianne Neifert, M.D., with Anne Price and Nancy Dana.** Move over Dr. Spock! Here comes Dr. Mom—the up-and-coming authority on child rearing! This indispensible reference covers every aspect of parenting from conception to age five, including: understanding medical symptoms, discipline, daycare, non-sexist child rearing and much more! (148509—$4.95)

☐ **TEACH YOUR BABY TO SLEEP THROUGH THE NIGHT by Charles E. Schaefer, Ph.D. and Michael R. Petronko, Ph.D.** The extraordinary Crying Baby Clinic program that solves you child's sleep problems in one week or less! "Essential facts and plausible advice to parents who are grappling with a child's sleep problems."—*Parenting* (156080—$3.95)

*Price slightly higher in Canada

Buy them at your local

bookstore or use coupon

on next page for ordering.

⊘ SIGNET (0451)

HELP YOURSELF—TO BETTER HEALTH!

- ☐ **FEEDING THE HUNGRY HEART: The Experience of Compulsive Eating by Geneen Roth.** Roth, once a compulsive overeater and self-starver, broke free from the destructive cycle of compulsive eating, and went on to help other women do the same. Those women are all here in this inspiring guide to show others that the battle against a hunger that goes deeper than a need for food *can be won.* "Amid all the diet books there is one—this one—that is different ... offers hope and inspiration." —*West Coast Review of Books* (158253—$4.50)*

- ☐ **SEEING SOLUTIONS by Barbara Ardinger, Ph.D.** Witness the power of your mind ... learn to use positive mental images to release unwanted thoughts and emotions and overcome stress, frustration, and anxiety. This step-by-step program will enable you to visualize your life as you want it to be—and make that vision a reality. (160096—$3.95)

- ☐ **KICKING YOUR STRESS HABITS: A Do-It-Yourself Guide for Coping With Stress by Donald A. Tubesing, Ph.D.** The 10-step program for getting rid of unhealthy stress, including: how to develop stress-managing skills; how to replace anxiety-producing attitudes with positive views; and how to break loose from a stressful lifestyle. (118340—$2.95)

- ☐ **FEELING GOOD: The New Mood Therapy by David D. Burns, M.D. Preface by Aaron T. Beck, M.D.** The clinically proven, drug-free treatment for depression, from the University of Pennsylvania School of Medicine. (158873—$4.95)*

- ☐ **EAT TO SUCCEED by Dr. Robert Haas.** In this groundbreaking book, the author of the #1 bestselling EAT TO WIN demonstrates how Ivan Lendl, Don Johnson, Cher and other celebrities have successfully used the revolutionary Haas Maximum Performance program and the Haas Maximum Weight Loss Plan. "Maximize alertness, unleash creativity and boost your energy and endurance."—*New York Post* (400887—$4.95)

*Prices slightly higher in Canada

Buy them at your local bookstore or use this convenient coupon for ordering.

NEW AMERICAN LIBRARY
P.O. Box 999, Bergenfield, New Jersey 07621
Please send me the books I have checked above. I am enclosing $_____
(please add $1.00 to this order to cover postage and handling). Send check or money order—no cash or C.O.D.'s. Prices and numbers are subject to change without notice.

Name_____

Address_____

City _____ State _____ Zip Code _____

Allow 4-6 weeks for delivery.
This offer, prices and numbers are subject to change without notice.

ⓢ SIGNET   (0451)

FOOD FOR THOUGHT

☐ **ARE YOU HUNGRY? by Jane R. Hirschmann and Lela Zaphiropoulos.** If your child drives you crazy at the dinner table, this completely new approach to raising children free of food and weight problems will demystify the myths and misconceptions about nutrition and help you start your child on a lifetime pattern of healthy eating. "Must reading for anyone who has ever had a feeding problem with a child."—American Library Association   (145135—$3.95)

☐ **LET'S STAY HEALTHY: A Guide to Lifelong Nutrition by Adelle Davis, edited and expanded by Ann Gildroy. Foreword by Leonard Lustgarten, M.D.** The wealth of advice and information in this definitive guide by America's most acclaimed nutritionist will serve as an essential aid in helping you formulate your own personal plan for lifelong vitality through good nutrition.   (119983—$4.95)

☐ **LET'S EAT RIGHT TO KEEP FIT by Adelle Davis.** Sensible, practical advice from America's foremost nutrition authority as to what vitamins, minerals and food balances you require; and the warning signs of diet deficiencies.
            (155505—$4.95)

☐ **LET'S COOK IT RIGHT by Adelle Davis.** For the first time in paperback, and completely revised and updated, the celebrated cookbook dedicated to good health, good sense and good eating. Contains 400 easy-to-follow, basic recipes, a table of equivalents and an index.
            (154614—$4.95)*

☐ **LET'S GET WELL by Adelle Davis.** America's most celebrated nutritionist shows how the proper selection of foods and supplements can hasten recovery from illness.   (154630—$4.95)*

☐ **LET'S HAVE HEALTHY CHILDREN by Adelle Davis.** America's most famous food expert gives the vital nutritional dos and don'ts for the expectant mother, babies, and growing children.   (154622—$4.95)

*Prices slightly higher in Canada

Buy them at your local bookstore or use this convenient coupon for ordering.

NEW AMERICAN LIBRARY
P.O. Box 999, Bergenfield, New Jersey 07621
Please send me the books I have checked above. I am enclosing $_____
(please add $1.00 to this order to cover postage and handling). Send check or money order—no cash or C.O.D.'s. Prices and numbers are subject to change without notice.

Name_____

Address_____

City _____ State _____ Zip Code _____

Allow 4-6 weeks for delivery.
This offer, prices and numbers are subject to change without notice.

There's an epidemic with 27 million victims. And no visible symptoms.

It's an epidemic of people who can't read.

Believe it or not, 27 million Americans are functionally illiterate, about one adult in five.

The solution to this problem is you... when you join the fight against illiteracy. So call the Coalition for Literacy at toll-free **1-800-228-8813** and volunteer.

Volunteer Against Illiteracy. The only degree you need is a degree of caring.

THIS AD PRODUCED BY MARTIN LITHOGRAPHERS
A MARTIN COMMUNICATIONS COMPANY